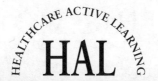

HEALTHCARE ACTIVE LEARNING

HAL

CONTEMPORARY SOCIAL POLICY

Start date

Target completion date

Tutor for this topic

Contact number

USING THIS WORKBOOK

The workbook is divided into 'Sessions', covering specific subjects.

In the introduction to each learning pack there is a learner profile to help you assess your current knowledge of the subjects covered in each session.

Each session has clear learning objectives. They indicate what you will be able to achieve or learn by completing that session.

Each session has a summary to remind you of the key points of the subjects covered.

Each session contains text, diagrams and learning activities that relate to the stated objectives.

It is important to complete each activity, making your own notes and writing in answers in the space provided. **Remember this is your own workbook—you are allowed to write on it**.

Now try an example activity.

ACTIVITY

This activity shows you what happens when cells work without oxygen. This really is a physical activity, so please only try it if you are fully fit.

First, raise one arm straight up in the air above your head, and let the other hand rest by your side. Clench both fists tightly, and then open out your fingers wide. Repeat this at the rate of once or twice a second. Try to keep clenching both fists at the same rate. Keep going for about five minutes, and record what you observe.

Stop and rest for a minute. Then try again, with the opposite arm raised this time. Again, record your observations.

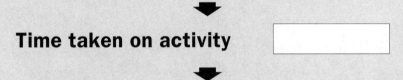

Suggested timings are given for each activity. These are only a guide. You may like to note how long it took you to complete this activity, as it may help in planning the time needed for working through the sessions.

Time taken on activity

Time management is important. While we recognise that people learn at different speeds, this pack is designed to take 20 study hours (your tutor will also advise you). You should allocate time during each week for study.

Take some time now to identify likely periods that you can set aside for study during the week.

Mon	Tues	Wed	Thurs	Fri	Sat	Sun
am						
pm						
eve						

At the end of the learning pack, there is a learning review to help you assess whether you have achieved the learning objectives.

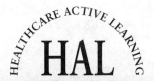

CONTEMPORARY
SOCIAL POLICY

Louise Ackers BSc. Econ MA

Senior Lecturer Social Policy, University of Plymouth

Jan Fordham BA MA

Open Learning Associates

THE OPEN LEARNING FOUNDATION

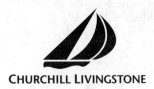

CHURCHILL LIVINGSTONE

NEW YORK EDINBURGH LONDON MADRID MELBOURNE SAN FRANCISCO AND TOKYO 1995

CHURCHILL LIVINGSTONE
Medical Division of Pearson Professional UK Limited

Distributed in the United States of America by Churchill
Livingstone Inc., 650 Avenue of the Americas, New York,
N.Y. 10011, and by associated companies, branches and
representatives throughout the world.

First published 1995

ISBN 0 443 05360 X

British Library of Cataloguing in Publication Data.
A catalogue record for this book is available from the
British Library.

Library of Congress Catalouging in Publication Data.
A catalogue record for this book is available from the
Library of Congress.

Produced through Longman Malaysia,

For The Open Learning Foundation

Director of Programmes: Leslie Mapp
Series Editor: Robert Adams
Programmes Manager: Kathleen Farren
Design and Production: Steve Moulds

For Churchill Livingstone

Project Manager: Valerie Burgess
Project Development Editor: Mairi McCubbin
Design Direction: Judith Wright
Sales Promotion Executive: Maria O'Connor

Contents

OPEN LEARNING FOUNDATION TEAM MEMBERS

Writer: Louise Ackers BSc. Econ MA
Senior Lecturer Social Policy
University of Plymouth

Editor: Jan Fordham BA MA
Open Learning Associates
London

Reviewer: Saul Becker BA MA CQSW PhD
Senior Lecturer in Social Policy
Department of Social Sciences
Loughborough University

Series Editor: Robert Adams
OLF Programme Head,
Social Work and Health and Nursing,
University of Humberside

THE OPEN LEARNING FOUNDATION

Higher education has grown considerably in recent years. As well as catering for more students, universities are facing the challenge of providing for an increasingly diverse student population. Students have a wider range of backgrounds and previous educational qualifications. There are greater numbers of mature students. There is a greater need for part-time courses and continuing education and professional development programmes.

The Open Learning Foundation helps over 20 member institutions meet this growing and diverse demand – through the production of high-quality teaching and learning materials, within a strategy of creating a framework for more flexible learning. It offers member institutions the capability to increase their range of teaching options and to cover subjects in greater breadth and depth.

It does not enrol its own students. Rather, The Open Learning Foundation, by developing and promoting the greater use of open and distance learning, enables universities and others in higher education to make study more accessible and cost-effective for individual students and for business through offering more choice and more flexible courses.

Formed in 1990, the Foundation's policy objectives are to:

- improve the quality of higher education and training

- increase the quantity of higher education and training

- raise the efficiency of higher education and training delivery.

In working to meet these objectives, The Open Learning Foundation develops new teaching and learning materials, encourages and facilitates more and better staff development, and promotes greater responsiveness to change within higher education institutions. The Foundation works in partnership with its members and other higher education bodies to develop new approaches to teaching and learning.

In developing new teaching and learning materials, the Foundation has:

- a track record of offering customers a swift and flexible response

- a national network of members able to provide local support and guidance

- the ability to draw on significant national expertise in producing and delivering open learning

- complete freedom to seek out the best writers, materials and resources to secure development.

Other titles in this series

Physiology

Genetics

Biochemistry

Experimental Research 1

Experimental Research 2

Descriptive Statistics

Legal Aspects of Health Care

INTRODUCTION

This unit seeks to increase your awareness of the extent to which social policy affects all of us in our everyday personal and working lives. It builds on your knowledge by considering substantive areas of social policy, in particular policies on health, community care and housing, and encourages you to think more broadly about the interrelationships between different aspects of social policy and the range of providers of welfare in society.

As you work through the unit, you will be introduced to some of the debates that have taken place within social policy as a discipline and consider the various political perspectives that have informed social policy developments. We shall look, for example, at the implications of the shift towards a greater reliance on the private, voluntary and informal sectors for the role of the state in the provision of social welfare. Finally, we shall consider the implications of these debates for health and social care professionals, particularly in terms of their role in the definition of need and its implications for dependency.

As you work through this unit, you will come across a number of activities which are designed to provide a guide for your learning. A time allowance has been included for each activity, but you should only regard it as a very rough estimate of how long it will take you to complete it. Don't be concerned if the activity takes more or less time than indicated.

Session One outlines the scope and functions of social policy and introduces the main sectors involved in welfare provision, exploring the ways in which different aspects of social policy interact to affect our lives, both personally and professionally.

Session Two focuses on health as a key issue in social policy. It examines the evidence of deep-rooted inequalities in health in the UK and considers the way in which different aspects of social policy impinge on the health of the population. It also examines the potential contribution of the Health of the Nation initiative in reducing these inequalities.

Session Three considers the contribution of the four main sectors involved in the implementation of social policy through the mixed economy of welfare – the statutory, private, voluntary and informal sectors – and explores their role under the provisions of the NHS and Community Care Act 1990.

Session Four examines the role of the statutory sector by exploring the ideologies of the two dominant political parties in the UK: the Conservative and Labour parties.

Session Five explores the growing role of the private sector in the provision of social welfare by focusing on housing and health, two areas in which the shift towards private provision has become particularly evident.

Session Six focuses on the role of the voluntary sector in meeting welfare needs, exploring the concept of altruism and assessing the growing importance of voluntarism within contemporary social policy.

Session Seven considers the role of the informal sector and the desirability and feasibility of an increasing reliance on the family as the primary provider of care. It explores the costs and benefits of informal care and potential constraints on further expansion of this sector.

Session Eight draws together your work on this unit by exploring the concept of need. It discusses the problems inherent in defining needs and examines how the ways in which needs are defined affect the experiences of those who are considered to be 'in need'.

LEARNING PROFILE

Below is a list of anticipated learning outcomes for each session in this unit. You can use it to assess your current level of knowledge and identify key areas on which you particularly need to focus. The learning profile is not intended to cover all the points discussed in each session, but provides a framework for you to decide how the unit can help you develop a fuller understanding of contemporary social policy.

For each of the learning outcomes listed below, tick the box that corresponds most closely to the point you feel you are at now. This will provide you with an assessment of your current knowledge, understanding and confidence in the areas that you will study in this unit. There is a similar exercise to complete at the end of the unit to help you review what you have learned.

	Not at all	Partly	Quite well	Very well
Session One				
I can:				
• define social policy	☐	☐	☐	☐
• outline three main perspectives on the functions of social policy	☐	☐	☐	☐
• identify the key sectors involved in welfare provision	☐	☐	☐	☐
• distinguish between the ways in which different socio-economic groups benefit most from the welfare state.	☐	☐	☐	☐
Session Two				
I can:				
• identify factors contributing to overall improvements in health in the UK	☐	☐	☐	☐
• summarise the evidence for the persistence of inequalities in health	☐	☐	☐	☐
• outline the major explanations for inequalities in health	☐	☐	☐	☐

	Not at all	Partly	Quite well	Very well

Session Two *continued*

- discuss the potential contribution of the Health of the Nation initiative to a reduction in inequalities in health.

| | ☐ | ☐ | ☐ | ☐ |

Session Three

I can:

- describe the roles of the four main sectors in the mixed economy of welfare

| | ☐ | ☐ | ☐ | ☐ |

- outline the provisions of the NHS and Community Care Act 1990

| | ☐ | ☐ | ☐ | ☐ |

- identify the providers of community care services in my local area.

| | ☐ | ☐ | ☐ | ☐ |

Session Four

I can:

- identify examples of social policy that reflect specific political ideologies

| | ☐ | ☐ | ☐ | ☐ |

- outline Conservative Party ideology on the role of the statutory sector

| | ☐ | ☐ | ☐ | ☐ |

- outline Labour Party ideology on the role of the statutory sector

| | ☐ | ☐ | ☐ | ☐ |

- discuss the advantages and disadvantages of universal and selective welfare provision.

| | ☐ | ☐ | ☐ | ☐ |

Session Five

I can:

- assess the impact of the shift towards private sector provision on the role of the state

| | ☐ | ☐ | ☐ | ☐ |

- identify the advantages and disadvantages of the emphasis on home-ownership in contemporary housing policy

| | ☐ | ☐ | ☐ | ☐ |

- discuss the implications of the growth in private heath care and the introduction of the internal market to the NHS for consumer choice, the quality of services and equality of access.

| | ☐ | ☐ | ☐ | ☐ |

	Not at all	Partly	Quite well	Very well

Session Six

I can:

- describe the range and scope of voluntary sector involvement in the provision of welfare

| | ☐ | ☐ | ☐ | ☐ |

- review some ideas and ideologies underpinning the expansion of the voluntary sector, in particular the notion of altruism or giving freely to others

| | ☐ | ☐ | ☐ | ☐ |

- assess the role of voluntarism and its place within social policy

| | ☐ | ☐ | ☐ | ☐ |

- suggest areas where voluntary sector involvement may be most appropriate.

| | ☐ | ☐ | ☐ | ☐ |

Session Seven

I can:

- identify the main categories of task undertaken by carers

| | ☐ | ☐ | ☐ | ☐ |

- discuss the advantages and disadvantages of informal and institutional care

| | ☐ | ☐ | ☐ | ☐ |

- discuss the significance of the gender of carers in determining the level of support provided

| | ☐ | ☐ | ☐ | ☐ |

- recognise potential constraints on the expansion of the informal sector.

| | ☐ | ☐ | ☐ | ☐ |

Session Eight

I can:

- discuss need as a relative concept

| | ☐ | ☐ | ☐ | ☐ |

- suggest why the way in which needs are defined has important implications for social policy

| | ☐ | ☐ | ☐ | ☐ |

- discuss how the definitions of need adopted by health and social care professionals can affect the experiences of those for whom they care.

| | ☐ | ☐ | ☐ | ☐ |

SESSION ONE

What is social policy?

Introduction

This first session encourages you to think about what you already know about social policy in the context of your own everyday work and personal life. It will not provide you with a single definition of social policy, but will introduce a range of ideas about what it is and what its functions are – or should be. By the time you have completed the unit, you should be aware of the complexity and far-reaching effects of social policy as well as the importance of recognising its broad relationship with other areas of government policy.

Session objectives

When you have completed this session, you should be able to:

● define social policy

● outline three main perspectives on the functions of social policy

● identify the key sectors involved in welfare provision

● distinguish between the ways in which different socio-economic groups benefit most from the welfare state.

Your thoughts on social policy

To help you begin to think about the role of social policy in contemporary society, the first activity asks you to think about what the term actually means.

ACTIVITY 1   ALLOW 5 MINUTES

What do you understand by the term 'social policy'? Note down the first five things that come to mind.

1

2

3

4

5

Commentary

Below are some of the comments that people typically make in response to the question 'What is social policy?'

'It's what social workers do. It's about helping people.'

'Social policy is to do with unemployment benefit, old age pensions, the NHS and so on.'

'Is it the same thing as sociology?'

'Something to do with the government.'

'It's all about politics and winning elections.'

These responses illustrate how people often have a rather hazy understanding of the meaning of social policy, even though they may recognise how it directly affects their lives. In fact, the term 'social policy' is conventionally used to describe government policy and the provision of services in six main areas:

- welfare benefits, such as social security and pensions

- unemployment

- the National Health Service (NHS)

- the personal social services

- education and training

- housing.

You may already have come across introductory textbooks such as *Introduction to Social Administration in Britain* (Brown, 1990) that deal with social policy in this way, with a chapter devoted to each of these issues.

In practice, however, social policy plays a significant role in our working and personal lives in ways that are much more complex and far-reaching than this simple division into six social policy areas might suggest. These areas are not separate and unrelated and a key theme of this unit is the way in which they interact – both with each other and with other areas of public policy, such as economic policy. Government policy on social security and the level of benefits, for example, affects recipients' housing situation with more generous benefits enabling them to afford higher levels of rent and perhaps avoid rent or mortgage arrears and homelessness. Government policy promoting home-ownership, which has been the focus of housing policy for the past twenty years, is affected by and affects economic policies, particularly those concerned with interest rates. The level of direct taxation (income tax) helps to determine the income people have available to spend on goods and services, while the level of indirect taxation, such as VAT, helps to determine the cost of those goods and services. Changes in fiscal policy determining both direct and indirect taxation may thus increase or decrease people's income which, in turn, has a major impact on the kind of housing they can afford and even on their health since it affects the amount of money that a household can devote to necessities such as food and heating. Conversely, the amount of money that the government can spend on implementing its social policies is directly related to the level of taxation which funds government spending. Other areas of government policy, such as industrial policy, also have an impact on social policy; increases in heavy manufacturing industry in a particular region, for example, might lead to higher levels of pollution with a consequent need for increased expenditure on health care.

The next activity asks you to reflect on these relationships further by considering the interaction between different aspects of social policy.

ACTIVITY 2   ALLOW 5 MINUTES

Note down two ways in which people's health might be improved by changes in housing and education policy.

1

2

Commentary

Health problems such as hypothermia, respiratory infections and stress are exacerbated by damp and ill-heated housing, overcrowding and homelessness, and childhood accidents are more common in high-rise flats and areas of poor housing that lack adequate facilities for play provision. The proportion of dwellings lacking basic amenities or being classified as unfit for human habitation has fallen dramatically with the post-war slum clearance programme, the renovation of local authority housing and the introduction of home improvement grants. Nevertheless, the 1991 English House Condition Survey revealed that about a million homes were unfit for human habitation and that nearly half a million lacked a basic amenity such as hot water or a toilet (Department of the Environment, 1993). Poor quality housing is concentrated particularly in urban areas, village centres and isolated rural areas; inner London, for example, has the highest proportion (16%) of dwellings in the 'worst' condition, as defined by the Department of the Environment (Central Statistical Office, 1994a). In 1993, 291 local authorities received no funds from central government for the management, maintenance and improvement of council homes, even though council housing contributed £722 million to the exchequer (Bayley, 1993). A change in policy permitting local authorities to invest more revenue from the sale of council homes in building new, low-rise housing stock and an increase in funds for renovation would result in the wider availability of good quality housing and could therefore be expected to have a significant effect on residents' health.

Education obviously plays an important role in health promotion. In an attempt to reduce the incidence of adolescent pregnancy and HIV/AIDS, for example, sex education has been introduced into the national curriculum and school nutrition education and anti-smoking campaigns are increasingly being focused on children who are particularly vulnerable to advertising that encourages them to adopt unhealthy lifestyles. In addition, healthy schools are seen as a key area for action in *The Health of the Nation: A strategy for health in England* in which the Department of Health (1992) stated its intention to establish a pilot network of health promoting schools which 'will develop, and assess the effectiveness of, strategies for changing and shaping pupils' patterns of behaviour, with the aim of safeguarding their long-term health.'

Education can also affect health in less direct ways. The expansion of government-funded training programmes for school-leavers and unemployed people, coupled with the growth in the number of places in further and higher education, is designed to reduce unemployment and increase people's income potential, both of which could result in improvements in health status.

It is thus important to recognise the relationship both between different areas of social policy and, in turn, with 'non-social' government policies because of the far-reaching effects of social policy in all areas of life.

The functions of social policy

Given that social policy has such an important influence on our lives, with the government being heavily involved in its provision, a fundamental question which then presents itself is, what are the functions of social policy? Why should the government or other agencies or sectors provide services such as housing or health services?

There are many different views about the role that social policy should play in society. Let us start by considering three of the main perspectives, which see its function as being to:

- meet need and/or prevent poverty

- promote equality, or at least equality of opportunity

- compensate for 'diswelfares' (or the social costs of industrial change).

Meeting need and preventing poverty

The importance of meeting need and preventing or reducing poverty is accepted by all political parties. They vary, however, in the way in which they define poverty. For many politicians on the right of the political spectrum, the role of social policy is to provide a safety-net to prevent people falling below certain *absolute* or minimum standards. We shall return to the question of who decides the level at which these standards should be set when we consider the issue of 'need' in Session Eight. Labour and Liberal Democrat politicians typically adopt a broader view of poverty, seeing it as a *relative* concept linked to prevailing living standards in that society. For them, the objective of preventing poverty is closely linked to that of promoting equality and social justice.

The view that the role of social policy is to act as a safety-net is based on the premise that there are two natural or socially-given channels through which an individual's needs are properly met – the private market and the family. Only when these break down should social welfare institutions come into play, and then only temporarily. This view has been termed the residual welfare model of social policy by Titmuss (1974).

This model sees the role of the government in the provision of welfare as being limited to meeting the needs only of those who can prove themselves to be in poverty or in need. Such proof typically requires some form of means test to assess any income and savings that applicants might have. They may also have to prove themselves to be deserving in the sense that their poverty or need is not their own fault by demonstrating, for example, that they are actively seeking work or that their homelessness is not intentional – that they had not failed to pay their rent or moved out of their parents' house voluntarily.

Supporters of the residual model argue that it is necessary to restrict welfare provision in this way in order to avoid unnecessary public expenditure and to limit the growth of what some Conservative politicians have referred to as the 'something for nothing society'.

As we shall see in Session Four, critics of this model argue that requiring people to prove their poverty, by undergoing extensive means tests and checks on their personal lives, often deters many people who are genuinely in need from applying for assistance. It has been estimated, for instance, that only 67% of elderly people claim the benefits to which they are entitled (Hill, 1990). Similarly, a survey conducted by the Policy Studies Institute (1993) found that although the take-up of family credit was higher than the official target set by the government in 1988, only 64% of the low-income families entitled to it were actually claiming it.

Promoting equality of opportunity

Advocates of the view that the function of social policy is to promote equality of opportunity argue that the state plays an important role in looking after the collective interests of society as a whole and that poverty in old age or inequalities between groups of people are problems that should properly be addressed by the government and not left to individuals to resolve. Most Labour and Liberal Democrat politicians would argue that social policy has a redistributive role: that is, that one of its main functions is to redistribute wealth and income via taxation in the form of welfare benefits and services. As such, for example, the state should ensure that all citizens have equal access to high quality education and an equal standard of health care, irrespective of their ability to pay. This means more than simply ensuring that every child has a place in a school or that every person has access to free health care. It might, for example, also involve taking positive action to provide 'compensatory education' for children living in deprived urban areas by providing extra places in nursery schools or additional teachers in primary schools, as in the Educational Priority Areas established in 1968 following the publication of the Plowden Report (1967) on primary schools.

In order to promote equality of opportunity, therefore, redistribution is required between different social groups: from the rich to the poor through differential rates of taxation to reduce inequalities in income, for example, or from able-bodied people to disabled people through programmes encouraging employers to recruit people with disabilities. It covers the duration of our lifespan, with children and elderly people likely to consume a greater proportion of welfare resources and people in their middle years contributing disproportionately.

Legislation may be necessary in the area of social policy in order to promote greater equality and control discriminatory behaviour. The Sex Discrimination Act 1975 and the Race Relations Act 1976 mark an important step in this direction. This legislation exists to ensure equal opportunity in society by preventing people, mainly employers, from making decisions about other people on the grounds of their gender or ethnic origin. The following activity asks you to think about the role of this kind of legislation and to consider the benefits and disadvantages of this form of social intervention.

ACTIVITY 3
ALLOW 30 MINUTES

Find out if there is an equal opportunities policy in your place of work, or in the college in which you are studying. Try to obtain a copy and summarise its main points. Why do you think we need policies of this kind?

If you are unable to locate an equal opportunities policy, read the policy of the University of Plymouth (1993) which has been reproduced as *Resource 1*.

Commentary

The strongest argument in favour of policies to overcome inequalities is that discrimination is wasteful of the talent of groups such as women, black people and people with disabilities and that society needs to make effective use of their energies and abilities, particularly at a time when there are skills shortages in specific areas. In addition, it is argued, permitting discrimination promotes social injustice and is therefore morally wrong. The state thus has a responsibility to play a leading role in preventing or reducing the incidence of injustices of this kind.

On the other hand, it is forcefully argued on the right of the political spectrum that it is not the job of the government to legislate for morality and that equal opportunities legislation can prove costly to employers; this may damage their competitive edge and make them less profitable as a result. This was certainly the view articulated by the Conservative government when it opted out of the Social Chapter of the Maastricht Treaty. It rejected, for example, the extension of maternity rights to part-time workers and workers who had worked for less than two years with a particular company on the grounds that it would put small businesses at a competitive disadvantage. Some leading Conservatives have also argued against the provisions on maternity rights on the grounds that it would encourage more women with young children to go out to work, which conflicts with their view of what good 'mothering' is all about and, paradoxically, denying legislation in this area on the grounds of morality. In September 1994, the government also rejected the extension of unpaid paternity leave to employees even though it was accepted by all other countries in the European Union.

Compensating for 'diswelfares'

The third main perspective on the function of social policy is that it should compensate for the social costs or 'diswelfares' of economic, technological and social change. A diswelfare might be described as some kind of disadvantage or loss experienced by an individual or a group of people as a result of another policy. So, for example, a decision by the government to promote the production of nuclear power in the interests of society as a whole might mean that a small number of people suffer disproportionately because of where they live and work. In 1992, for example, evidence was submitted to court which suggested that children living in the area around the Sellafield nuclear power station experience higher rates of leukaemia though, in its final judgement, the court did not find this link to be conclusive. For proponents of the 'compensating for diswelfares' view, social policy should have a compensatory function in such cases, with special provision being made for monitoring the health of the local population and treating those affected.

Similarly, the introduction of new technology in order to maintain international competitiveness and profitability may be in the general interest of the economy and society as a whole. One unintended consequence of investment in technological change, however, may be an increase in unemployment in some areas of work, such as has occurred in the car industry and other parts of the manufacturing sector. How far does society have a responsibility to compensate those who become unemployed as a consequence through special retraining schemes or regional development aid?

Policy implementation and the provision of social welfare

We have seen that different views exist about the appropriate function of social policy within society. Such views not only determine the nature of the social policies developed by government, but also raise questions about their implementation and responsibility for the provision of social welfare. In particular, there are different views about what the respective roles of the government, the private sector, employers, voluntary organisations and the family should be.

Traditionally, the study of social policy has been confined to the statutory sector: that is, to direct provision by central and local government in areas such as social services, welfare benefits, state education, public housing and the National Health Service. Yet, in order to understand the role of social policy in society and how people experience it, we need to go beyond this rather limited approach.

In an influential essay entitled *The Social Division of Welfare*, Titmuss (1955) stressed the importance of three welfare systems, which he termed:

- social welfare: provision by the government

- occupational welfare: provision by employers

- fiscal welfare: provision via the taxation system.

Some understanding of the contribution of each of these aspects of welfare is necessary in order to appreciate the full impact of social policy. To focus solely on the statutory sector within the welfare state can result in a very misleading impression of social policy being inherently benevolent and redistributive: in other words, disproportionately benefiting the 'poor'. An analysis that takes full account of all three dimensions and of the interaction between them gives a very different impression of the redistributive effects of social policy. Let us consider for a moment the issue of pensions. In 1992–93, over 9.9 million people were receiving state retirement pensions from the state, with a further 340,000 receiving a widow's pension (Central Statistical Office, 1994a). Mrs X might receive only the state pension while her neighbour, Ms Y, might receive the same state pension plus an occupational pension from her employer or a private pension from a scheme to which she was encouraged to subscribe through various tax relief incentives. In 1992, 62% of male full-time employees, 55% of female full-time employees and 19% of female part-time employees were members of their current employer's pension scheme. Membership of private pension schemes was 27%, 21% and 12% respectively (OPCS, 1994).

In order to understand the full impact of social policy, we might also want to add to Titmuss's categories and take into account the contribution of three further welfare systems:

- private welfare: provision by the private sector

- voluntary welfare: provision by charitable and voluntary organisations such as Help the Aged or MENCAP

- informal welfare: provision within the home, usually by the family.

To continue with our example of pensions, Mrs Z might receive additional support from a private insurance policy, from her children or from a voluntary organisation established to assist the widows of, for instance, ex-police officers or war veterans. We can see from this example that, in relation to pensions policy at least, there are many different providers of welfare. Whilst the state retirement pension itself may constitute a form of redistribution, the distributional effects are far more complex when we also consider the impact of other forms of pension, some of which are state-subsidised.

Similarly, housing is provided by a very broad range of agencies, some of which receive support from the government. Housing is provided directly by local government in the form of council housing, but also indirectly through housing benefit, which enables many tenants in local authority and privately rented accommodation to claim back some or all of their rent. Government policies on mortgage interest tax relief and the sale of council homes have actively promoted home-ownership; by 1992, nearly two-thirds of the housing stock was owner-occupied and there were more than twice as many owner-occupied homes than in 1961, including nearly 1.5 million that had been purchased by council tenants. The private sector now dominates housebuilding, with companies such as Wimpey and Barratt building around 80% of the nation's new homes in 1992, including 38% of sheltered housing and other specialised homes for elderly people. The voluntary sector has an increasingly important role to play in housing, which is encouraged by government subsidies to housing associations through the Housing Corporation. By 1992, housing associations owned one in ten properties and built 44% of the new specialised properties for elderly people in 1992 (Central Statistical Office, 1994a). Some employers also play a role in the provision of housing; many banks, for example, subsidise employees' mortgages by offering low mortgage interest rates and members of the armed forces often benefit from 'tied' housing schemes. Other people choose, or are forced, to live with family or friends.

The second column in *Figure 1* below illustrates the scope of social policy in relation to housing by indicating the roles of the different welfare sectors. Initiatives subsidised by central or local government are marked with an asterisk. *Activity 4* is designed to encourage you to think about the roles played by different agencies in the provision of health care and about how they interact with each other.

	Housing	Health
Statutory welfare	Local authority housing* Housing benefit*	
Occupational welfare	Mortgage subsidy* Tied housing	
Fiscal welfare	Mortgage interest relief*	
Private welfare	Home ownership*	
Voluntary welfare	Housing associations*	
Informal welfare	Sharing with family or friends	

Figure 1: Roles of different welfare sectors

ACTIVITY 4 — ALLOW 10 MINUTES

Look at the second column in *Figure 1* which indicates the range of providers of housing. Then complete the third column in a similar way, this time focusing on health care. Indicate both the roles played by different agencies and the areas that are state-subsidised.

Commentary

The National Health Service clearly comes under the heading 'statutory welfare' as it represents services directly provided by the government. Tax incentives for older people to subscribe to private health insurance schemes are an example of fiscal welfare: that is, welfare promoted by the government through the taxation system. Occupational welfare includes benefits such as private health insurance for individual employees and the provision of occupational health facilities, workplace health education programmes and sports facilities. Voluntary provision includes the contribution of organisations such as the Cancer Relief Macmillan Fund, which provides nursing care for many people with cancer, the hospice movement which provides palliative and terminal care, and agencies such as the British Heart Foundation which are concerned with specific aspects of health and illness. Private health care includes the purchase by individuals of services to supplement or substitute for NHS provision, such as private health insurance, private dental treatment, private medical and nursing care at home, in residential care homes, nursing homes and hospital, as well as services such as chiropody and complementary therapies such as homeopathy or acupuncture. As we shall see in Session Seven, the informal sector is responsible for many areas of health care, from home care by family and friends to providing lifts to hospital and educating children about healthy living.

This is by no means an exhaustive list and you have probably suggested a number of other ways in which different agencies are involved in the provision of health care. You might like to repeat this activity using other social policy areas such as education or social services. This activity could form the basis for a group discussion.

Who benefits from social policy?

Having considered the different ways in which welfare is provided, it is possible to appreciate more clearly the role that social policy plays in all our lives and to consider who benefits most from the range of policies and welfare providers we have discussed. Many people who are in good health, have a job and own their own home may feel that social policy affects them very little – except that they have to pay taxes. However, it is possible to challenge the commonly-held view that, broadly speaking, there are those who benefit from social welfare and those who pay for it. The following activity encourages you to think about the different ways in which people benefit from social policy.

ACTIVITY 5 — ALLOW 5 MINUTES

List the various ways in which you feel that you and your family currently benefit from social policy.

Commentary

With some aspects of social policy, it is relatively easy to assess whether or not you benefit personally. If you receive child benefit or family credit, have children who go to the local state school or have recently had an operation in an NHS hospital, you will readily accept this as a tangible benefit to yourself and your family. If you own your own home, the government helps to subsidise the cost of your mortgage through tax relief. On the other hand, if you live in privately-rented accommodation, have no children, receive no grant for the course you are undertaking, have never claimed any social security benefits and are a member of a private health insurance scheme, you may feel that you do not benefit personally from government welfare provision. But think about ways in which you may benefit indirectly from areas of social policy that contribute to a more healthy and better-educated society and that, it could be argued, increase the overall standard of living in the UK as a result. Education and training programmes designed to promote higher levels of employment, for instance, may contribute to reduced levels of crime and delinquency and therefore benefit us all indirectly.

Le Grand (1982) has undertaken a considerable volume of research that suggests that it is, in fact, the middle classes who are the main beneficiaries of the welfare state and not, as is popularly perceived, the working classes. The next activity focuses on an article by Woolley and Le Grand (1990) which compares the impact of the welfare state on hypothetical working-class and middle-class families.

ACTIVITY 6   ALLOW 45 MINUTES

Read *Resource 2, The Ackroyds, the Osbornes and the Welfare State: The impact of the welfare state on two hypothetical families over their life-times* (Woolley and Le Grand, 1990).

Woolley and Le Grand argue that the redistributive effects of social policy are complex. On what grounds do they conclude that welfare state expenditure does not amount to a simple redistribution in favour of poorer members of society?

Commentary

Woolley and Le Grand acknowledge the difficulties of assessing the redistributive effects of the welfare state since the extent to which specific groups of services benefit working-class and middle-class families obviously varies according to their individual needs and circumstances. Nevertheless, although they use hypothetical families to illustrate their case, the life histories of the Ackroyds and the Osbornes are based on statistical data that reflect the life expectancy, number of children, education patterns, accommodation and recreation choices of 'typical' families in the two socio-economic groups. On this basis, Woolley and Le Grand argue that the welfare state, taken as a whole to include tax relief on private sector provision as well as direct expenditure by the statutory sector, does not simply redistribute welfare resources in favour of poorer sections of society.

Their study shows that direct expenditure on cash benefits, apart from retirement pensions, tends to benefit working-class families disproportionately. However, direct expenditure on pensions is greater for the middle classes, even where they do not receive tax relief on private pension schemes, largely because they have a longer life expectancy (we shall return to the relationship between inequalities in health and social class in Session Two). Similarly, expenditure on housing and education favours the middle classes since they are more likely to be owner-occupiers receiving mortgage interest tax relief, with children who remain at school beyond the age of sixteen and who go on to higher education.

As well as comparing typical spending on families such as the Ackroyds and Osbornes, Woolley and Le Grand examine the financial contributions that they make through taxation. The evidence they present suggests that, as might be expected, middle-income groups such as the Osbornes contribute to a greater extent through direct taxation. However, it is important to note that lower-income groups contribute to a greater extent through indirect taxation, including such elements as tobacco revenue.

In considering some of the ways in which the middle classes might benefit from welfare provision, you may recall that Titmuss (1955) highlighted the important contribution of occupational welfare. He referred to this as the 'concealed multiplier of occupational success': in other words, people's occupational success tends to be matched by increasing welfare privilege. The contribution of this sector is often overlooked by social policy analysts.

ACTIVITY 7   ALLOW 5 MINUTES

Try to identify at least two examples of occupational welfare as 'the concealed multiplier of occupational success'.

Commentary

In practice, the higher people's earnings or status are the more likely it is that their employer provides them with some form of welfare goods or benefits. If we look more closely at the issue of pensions, we find that three-quarters of full-time professional men and two-thirds of professional women interviewed in the 1992 General Household Survey (OPCS, 1994) belonged to an occupational pension scheme compared with 45% of men and 37% of women working full-time in unskilled manual work, although there were considerable variations between different kinds of employment. Employee benefits may also include subsidised mortgages or tied housing, subsidised meals or luncheon vouchers, a company car or a workplace day nursery which is so crucial in enabling many women to return to work. In the area of health care, many employees receive private health insurance and access to occupational health facilities. However, most of these benefits are more commonly available to higher status employees or white-collar workers, which effectively turns the argument that social policy is about meeting need on its head. For, in effect, the higher your income and the less need you have for welfare provision, the more likely you are to receive it in some form from your employer – and some of this may even be subsidised by the tax-payer.

Titmuss therefore argued the importance of taking occupational welfare into account in assessing the redistributional effects of welfare systems as it clearly challenges the view that the function of social policy is primarily to meet the needs of the poor.

In this introductory session, we have addressed a number of issues that are crucial to any understanding of contemporary social policy. Ginsburg (1993) presents a useful working definition that provides the context for our subsequent discussion of these issues:

> 'The terms "social policy" and "the welfare state" are virtually synonymous. They are conventionally used to describe government action in the fields of personal and family income, health care, housing, education and training, and personal "care" services. "Government action" embraces not only direct provision of benefits and services, but also the regulation and subsidy (including fiscal reliefs) of the various private forms of welfare. These latter include occupational welfare, provided by employers, welfare provided by for-profit, charitable, trade union, community, religious and other voluntary organizations, as well as that provided informally by family members, friends and neighbours. Clearly the boundaries of social policy extend into areas which are conventionally ascribed to "economic policy" (e.g. employment, industrial, monetary and fiscal policy) and other areas of public policy (e.g. immigration, law enforcement, industrial relations and penal policy).'

As you progress through the unit, you will be encouraged to assess the information and knowledge that you acquire in the light of this definition and the themes raised in this session. In particular, try to keep the following questions in mind.

1 What is the proper role of the state and to what extent should it be involved in the social and economic life of society? Should the state actively promote equality of access and opportunity through such interventions as positive action programmes? Or should its involvement be more limited, encouraging people to meet their needs through the family and the private sector?

2 How should welfare be provided? What should be the respective roles of the individual, the family, the voluntary sector, the private sector, occupational welfare and the statutory sector? Should the consumers of welfare be more involved in shaping the nature and allocation of welfare services? Do they have rights?

3 What kind of intervention or welfare provision is appropriate? Should welfare benefits and services be universally available, as of right, or should they be selective and subject to means testing?

Throughout the rest of this unit, we shall explore these issues in greater detail as we consider the major debates that are taking place within the field of social policy. In doing so, we hope that you will become more aware of the important role that social policy plays in all our lives and of its impact on you and those around you. In Session Two, we shall focus specifically on the area of health and how different aspects of social policy relate to inequalities in health.

Summary

1 Social policy covers six broad areas: welfare benefits, unemployment, health, social services, education and housing. These policy areas are interrelated and also relate to wider areas of public policy, particularly economic policy.

2 Three of the most influential perspectives on the functions of social policy are that it is:

- to meet need and prevent poverty
- to promote equality of opportunity
- to compensate for 'diswelfares'.

3 The statutory sector is not the sole source of welfare provision; the occupational, fiscal, private, voluntary and informal sectors all provide benefits and/or services.

4 Social policy is popularly thought to be concerned purely with meeting need and preventing poverty, but the middle classes benefit from the welfare state as much as, if not more than, the working classes.

Before you move on to Session Two, check that you have achieved the objectives given at the beginning of this session and, if not, review the appropriate sections.

Inequalities in health and social policy

Introduction

As the main provider of health care in the UK, the National Health Service has a statutory responsibility to provide equal access to health services that are free at the point of use. Yet inequalities in health persist in this country, as evidenced by differences in mortality and morbidity rates between social groups. In this session, we shall explore some of the theories that have been put forward to account for these inequalities and consider ways in which health is affected not only by access to health care, but also by lifestyle, social class, poverty and other aspects of social policy such as housing and employment as well as the wider economic structure. We shall also consider the impact that the health promotion initiative introduced by the Department of Health in its Health of the Nation strategy might have on inequalities in health.

Session objectives

When you have completed this session, you should be able to:

- identify factors contributing to overall improvements in health in the UK

- summarise the evidence for the persistence of inequalities in health

- outline the major explanations for inequalities in health

- discuss the potential contribution of the Health of the Nation initiative to a reduction in inequalities in health.

Health and the NHS

The establishment of the welfare state in the 1940s marked the culmination of over a century of social reform that attempted to reshape the Poor Law, first introduced in 1601 and remaining on the statute book until 1948, to the modern world. Its architect was William Beveridge whose influential report to government in 1942 had proposed a means by which the scourges of disease, want, squalor, ignorance and idleness could be eliminated. For Beveridge, 'the abolition of want requires a double redistribution of income through social insurance and by family needs' and his proposals included the introduction of family allowances, the establishment of the National Insurance system, the final abolition of the Poor Law and its replacement by the National Assistance scheme. Central to his proposals was the creation of a universal health service that, in the words of a government White Paper (Ministry of Health, 1944), would:

> ' ... ensure that in future every man and woman and child can rely on getting all the advice and treatment and care which they may need in matters of personal health; that what they get shall be the best medical and other facilities available; that their getting these shall not depend on whether they can pay for them, or on any other factor irrelevant to the real need – the real need being to bring the country's full resources to bear upon reducing ill-health and promoting good health in all its citizens ... '

The assurance that, for the first time, health care would be available to all on the basis of medical need rather than the ability to pay is widely regarded as one of the notable achievements of the twentieth century. Although the service initially focused largely on cure rather than prevention and services remained somewhat fragmented in the early years, the establishment of the National Health Service in

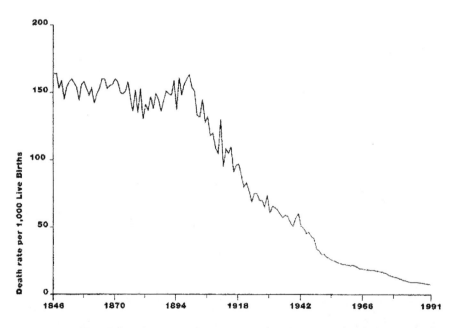

Figure 2: Infant mortality in the UK, 1846–1991 (Department of Health, 1992)

1948 contributed directly to a steady and significant improvement in the overall health of the British people, as illustrated by increases in life expectancy and the virtual eradication of diseases that were previously common, such as tuberculosis and poliomyelitis. A particularly graphic indicator of improved health is the continuing fall in the infant mortality rate – that is, the number of deaths of infants under one year of age per 1000 live births – which, by 1992, had fallen to 6.6 per 1000 from 59 per 1000 in 1940–42 (Central Statistical Office, 1994b). Yet, as *Figure 2* shows, the most dramatic reductions in infant mortality during the last hundred years occurred *before* the NHS was established. The following activity encourages you to think about the contribution of different aspects of social policy to the decline in infant mortality.

ACTIVITY 8   ALLOW 5 MINUTES

Note down at least three ways in which you think the NHS has contributed to the continuing fall in infant mortality rates. What other factors might also have helped to reduce the rate of infant deaths? You might find it interesting to talk to women of different generations in your family to compare their experiences of pregnancy and childbirth.

Commentary

A broad range of developments in medical technology and health service provision introduced since the establishment of the NHS have contributed to the fall in infant mortality. These include:

- free access to midwifery and obstetric care

- the expansion of antenatal and postnatal care, particularly by midwives and health visitors

- the shift from home to hospital deliveries, particularly after the publication of the Peel Report in 1970

- improved training in midwifery and obstetrics

- medical and technological advances, such as anaesthesia, blood transfusion, antibiotics, chorionic villus sampling, ultrasonography, amniocentesis and fetal monitoring

- free milk and vitamin supplements for expectant mothers and children under the age of five, introduced in 1940 but now restricted to certain groups, such as families receiving income support

- an expanded programme of immunisation for infants and children

- wider access to family planning, resulting in improved child spacing and smaller family sizes

- the recent reduction in the incidence of Sudden Infant Death Syndrome (cot-deaths) through the issuing of new guidance to parents on preventive measures.

The Health of the Nation (Department of Health, 1992) points to the potential for further reductions in infant mortality through health promotion programmes aimed at pregnant women and notes, in particular, the importance of initiatives to discourage women from smoking during pregnancy. Broader social policies such as the provision of maternity leave through the introduction of statutory maternity pay and maternity allowance have also promoted the health of the mother during late pregnancy and following birth and hence the health of the baby.

The dramatic fall in infant mortality in the UK in the century before the NHS was established suggests, however, that subsequent improvements cannot be attributed solely to free access to improved health care services. In his work, The Modern Rise of Population and the Role of Medicine (1976), McKeown argues that the main reasons for the decline in infant mortality rates and the improvement in health of the population as a whole are to be found in the improved social, economic and environmental conditions in which we all now live. While acknowledging the contribution of medical advances and improved service provision to better health, he suggests that these factors have been of only marginal importance compared with the effects of better housing, diet and working conditions and to wider developments in public and environmental health that have resulted in a safe water supply and sanitation system. Indeed, as Merret (1979) points out, one of the key impetuses for the development of public housing in the UK after the First World War arose from a concern by industrialists over the loss of working days, and hence profitability, as a result of workers' poor health.

Much of the improvement in the overall health of the population can thus be attributed to broader socio-economic factors rather than simply to the availability of better health care services through the NHS. The quality of health has, however, improved more for some sectors of the population than for others. So, despite the fact that people are generally much healthier now than only fifty years ago, the inequalities in health that existed then between different social groups remain with us today. We turn now to the issue of inequalities in health between different groups within society.

Inequalities in health

An important step in demonstrating the inequalities in health that exist between different social groups came with the publication of the Short Report on perinatal and neonatal mortality (Social Services Committee, 1980). The Committee observed that although the perinatal and neonatal mortality rates had improved considerably in England and Wales, they were twice as high in the lowest socio-economic classes as in the highest and that a significant number of children were surviving each year with severe 'handicaps' that were preventable. They concluded that the factors causing perinatal and neonatal mortality and handicap broadly divided into two interrelated categories:

- socio-economic factors, such as a lack of education, poverty, poor housing, poor nutrition, unplanned pregnancy, smoking and excess alcohol consumption

- medical factors, such as a lack of antenatal care, low birthweight, asphyxia during delivery or afterwards, congenital malformations and cerebral haemorrhage.

The Short Report was significant in pointing to the social and economic problems that lay at the root of some cases of infant mortality and morbidity, but it was the Black Report (Department of Health & Social Security, 1980) that first highlighted the extent of health inequalities in the UK. The report analysed inequalities between different social classes using the Registrar General's classification of socio-economic groups. This is based on various factors such as income, education, housing and employment and groups people into the following categories:

I   Professional (such as lawyers, doctors and accountants)

II   Intermediate (such as teachers, nurses and managers)

IIIN Skilled non-manual (such as typists and shop assistants)

IIIM Skilled manual (such as miners, bus drivers and cooks)

IV   Partly-skilled manual (such as farm workers and bus conductors)

V   Unskilled manual (such as cleaners and labourers).

The Black Report provided clear evidence of a relationship between an individual's social class and the likelihood of that individual experiencing ill-health. It demonstrated not only that inequalities in health existed, but also that they had widened in the previous decade or so. While overall mortality rates had declined for all groups, they had fallen at a slower pace amongst working-class people and the incidence of illness and ill-health was also greater among the lower socio-economic groups. The Report made 37 recommendations on ways of reducing inequalities in health, many of which addressed the underlying socio-economic causes. Of these, the most important were:

- the abolition of child poverty

- improvements in housing

- improvements in working conditions

- improved provision for disabled people

- a co-ordinated national and local government policy

- the establishment of a Health Development Council to plan and monitor the implementation of the policy recommendations.

In 1987, the Health Education Council (now the Health Education Authority) published *The Health Divide: Inequalities in health in the 1980s* (Whitehead, 1988) which reviewed many studies carried out since the publication of the Black Report in order to update the evidence on inequalities in health and assess the progress made in relation to its recommendations. Like the Black Report, it used the Registrar General's classifications of social class. *The Health Divide* supported the findings of the Black Report that health inequalities are largely related to an individual's class and concluded that they still persisted in the late 1980s. Amongst the many health inequalities that were found to exist, the following most clearly illustrate the relationship between ill-health and social class.

- Children born to group V families are twice as likely to die in their first year of life as children born to a group I family.

- The standardised mortality ratio (SMR) or the relative chances of death at any given age is twice as high for members of group V as for group I.

- Most of the major and minor killer diseases now affect the poorest occupational classes more than the rich.

- Not only do lower occupational groups have higher death rates, they also experience more sickness and ill-health throughout their lives.

- Health deteriorates more rapidly amongst elderly people in groups IV and V than in groups I and II.

As *Figures 3* and *4* show, these inequalities between different social classes exist from the moment of birth and tend to persist throughout life.

Differentials in mortality and morbidity rates are not simply found between social classes, however. Equally striking is the health gap between different parts of the country and, for some health conditions, between the sexes and different ethnic groups. In November 1993, for example, figures obtained from the Department of Health through a Parliamentary question by a Labour MP, Alan Milburn, showed that people are more likely to die prematurely if they live north of a line between the Wash and the Severn (Brindle, 1993a). The breakdown of expected and actual deaths in the 14 English health regions showed that six regions, representing the North and the Midlands, had 232,000 more deaths than expected in 1991 and eight, representing the South, had 235,000 fewer – the same pattern as in 1979. *Figure 5* shows the percentage difference between the number of expected and actual deaths by health region.

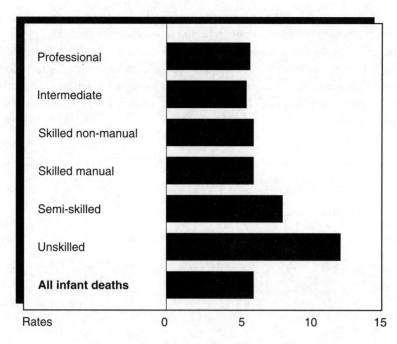

Figure 3: Infant mortality by social class of father, 1990
(Source: Central Statistical Office, 1993a)

Great Britain						Percentages and numbers	
	Prof- essional	Employers and managers	Inter- mediate	Skilled manual	Semi- skilled manual	Unskilled manual	Total
Condition group							
Musculoskeletal system	10.0	12.6	13.0	15.5	17.1	20.1	14.5
Heart and circulatory system	6.4	8.1	8.0	9.4	11.8	12.1	9.1
Respiratory system	5.2	5.2	6.8	6.4	7.2	9.6	6.4
Digestive system	2.1	3.3	4.0	3.9	4.8	5.0	3.8
Nervous system	2.5	2.1	3.1	2.7	2.9	4.4	2.8
Eye complaints	1.5	2.2	2.9	2.0	3.0	3.2	2.4
Ear complaints	1.9	1.4	1.9	2.7	2.5	3.1	2.2
All long-standing illness	29.1	32.5	34.9	37.0	41.6	47.8	36.5
Sample size (= 100%)(numbers)	1,164	3,557	4,065	5,987	3,190	981	19,562

Figure 4: Reported long-standing illness or disability by socio-economic group and condition group, 1989 (Source: Central Statistical Office, 1993a)

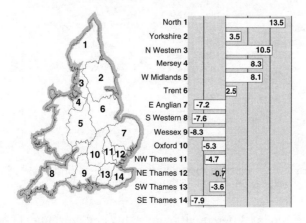

Figure 5: Regional divide: percentage difference between the number of expected and actual deaths (Source: Brindle, 1993a)

If you look more closely at the mortality rates for 1991 shown in *Figure 6*, you can see the variations between the English regional health authorities and between the four countries of the United Kingdom. You can also see that there are differences in the cause of death between the sexes, with men experiencing higher mortality rates for ischaemic heart disease, respiratory diseases, cancer, injuries and poisoning, and women having higher mortality rates for cerebrovascular disease and other causes.

| | All circulatory diseases | | | All respiratory diseases | | | All injuries and poisonings | | | | |
	Total	Ischaemic heart disease	Cerebro-vascular disease	Total	Bronchitis and allied conditions	Cancer	Total	Road traffic accidents	Suicides and open verdicts	All other causes	All causes
Males											
United Kingdom	509	331	105	126	20	301	46	13	18	137	1,117
Northern	581	386	123	139	22	336	45	14	17	145	1,245
Yorkshire	523	350	114	137	22	304	43	13	17	133	1,138
Trent	508	335	102	129	20	295	44	15	17	137	1,112
East Anglia	458	288	102	93	17	268	47	15	18	130	994
North West Thames	450	291	89	120	17	283	43	10	18	141	1,036
North East Thames	475	307	93	130	16	302	45	11	18	155	1,105
South East Thames	467	291	92	118	23	297	42	11	18	135	1,057
South West Thames	448	281	86	104	19	273	38	10	16	129	990
Wessex	448	288	93	93	15	282	40	13	18	134	998
Oxford	445	281	94	118	15	284	41	11	16	130	1.016
South Western	474	296	100	94	18	266	43	14	18	128	1.004
West Midlands	520	336	111	127	27	308	42	12	15	141	1,137
Mersey	534	353	109	144	20	336	44	11	15	144	1,200
North Western	559	371	113	146	29	323	51	11	21	144	1,221
England	495	320	102	121	21	297	43	12	17	137	1,093
Wales	524	349	106	127	24	294	48	13	19	131	1,122
Scotland	602	392	132	153	14	330	62	14	21	142	1,288
Northern Ireland	578	393	108	201	22	297	68	19	13	105	1,250
Females											
United Kingdom	526	266	166	127	13	266	25	5	6	181	1,125
Northern	600	324	184	139	15	290	26	6	5	201	1,255
Yorkshire	536	290	167	132	13	264	24	5	6	187	1,142
Trent	530	274	161	129	13	260	23	6	6	191	1,133
East Anglia	474	234	154	102	10	239	25	6	6	194	1,033
North West Thames	458	232	135	128	13	256	24	5	7	189	1,054
North East Thames	468	233	147	124	10	263	23	4	6	201	1,255
South East Thames	501	239	155	117	12	258	22	5	7	171	1,069
South West Thames	479	228	147	113	13	248	19	5	6	181	1,039
Wessex	479	230	164	96	9	241	22	6	6	189	1.025
Oxford	457	219	152	124	10	257	24	5	4	194	1.056
South Western	482	229	162	96	11	247	23	5	6	178	1.025
West Midlands	531	264	171	120	14	261	25	4	5	190	1,126
Mersey	552	291	163	156	15	280	19	4	6	187	1,192
North Western	592	306	185	145	19	273	28	5	6	182	1,219
England	513	258	161	123	13	260	23	5	6	188	1,106
Wales	531	273	166	120	15	263	27	4	5	170	1,110
Scotland	628	317	205	151	9	284	40	6	7	175	1,277
Northern Ireland	592	307	183	228	10	258	33	6	6	111	1,221

Rates per 100,000 population

Figure 6: Age-adjusted mortality rates by cause and sex, 1991
(Source: Central Statistical Office, 1993b)

There is evidence, too, of differentials in mortality and morbidity between ethnic groups. Some illnesses are largely confined to particular ethnic communities; sickle cell disease and thalassaemia, for example, are found in people of African,

Caribbean, Asian and Mediterranean origin. For other illnesses, however, there is not such a simple explanation. *Figure 7* shows the number of deaths and standardised mortality ratios for coronary heart disease (CHD) and stroke by country of birth in 1979–1983 in England and Wales. This indicates that men of Asian origin have a 36% higher death rate from CHD than their indigenous counterparts and that women have a 46% higher rate. They also have a higher death rate from stroke, although the difference is not so great as for the Afro-Caribbean population, where the death rates are 76% higher for men and 110% higher for women.

| | Coronary Heart Disease | | Stroke | |
	Numbers of deaths	SMRs	Numbers of deaths	SMRs
Men Aged 20-69				
All persons	69,248	100	3,746	100
Scotland	4,959	111	834	105
All Ireland	6,225	114	1,175	123
Indian subcontinent	3,410	136	645	153
Caribbean Commonwealth	669	45	419	176
African Commonwealth	400	113	103	163
Old Commonwealth	584	91	112	95
West Europe	717	77	97	62
East Europe	2,453	112	407	105
Republic of South Africa	165	90	31	93
United States	231	86	54	112
Women Aged 20-69				
All persons	69,248	100	32,037	100
Scotland	1,496	119	637	110
All Ireland	2,023	120	922	117
Indian subcontinent	798	146	347	125
Caribbean Commonwealth	214	76	316	210
African Commonwealth	62	97	58	139
Old Commonwealth	153	72	99	101
West Europe	376	81	163	73
East Europe	264	110	117	109
Republic of South Africa	59	73	42	112
United States	40	56	23	65

Figure 7: Deaths and standardised mortality ratios for coronary heart disease and stroke by country of birth, 1979–1983, England and Wales (Source: British Heart Foundation/Coronary Prevention Group, 1994)

You may find it interesting to read Chapter 2 of *The Health Divide* (Whitehead, 1988) which assesses patterns of health inequality in the late 1980s and to think about how it reflects your own experience of health and health care.

ACTIVITY 9 ALLOW **15** MINUTES

Note down your ideas on the reasons why inequalities in health persist in the 1990s, despite a general improvement in people's health.

Commentary

The studies cited by the Black Report and *The Health Divide* as well as subsequent research studies show there to be a clear association between ill-health and lower social class and, despite the variations between geographical regions, ethnic groups and the sexes, poverty appears to be the common factor. It is by no means clear, however, why this is so. There is no simple explanation for inequalities in health but, in the next section, we shall consider a number of factors that together give us some understanding of why people in lower social classes tend to experience poorer health than those in higher social classes.

Explanations for health inequalities

In 1985, the World Health Organization (WHO) Regional Office for Europe set a series of health targets to be achieved by member states by the year 2000. Central to these targets was the principle of equality: 'By the year 2000, the actual differences in health status between countries and between groups within countries should be reduced by at least 25%, by improving the health of disadvantaged nations and groups.' As WHO recognised, however, it is important to distinguish between equality in health care and equality in health:

> In terms of *health care*, the principle of social justice leads to 'equal access to available care, equal treatment for equal cases and equal quality of care.'

> In terms of *health*, 'ideally everyone should have the *same opportunity* to attain the highest level of health and, more pragmatically, none should be unduly disadvantaged.'

A logical starting point for an explanation of inequalities in health, then, is to consider whether people actually do have equal access to services, equal treatment and equal quality of care before exploring possible reasons why people may not have equal opportunities to attain or maintain good health.

Equal access for equal need

One possible explanation for the persistence of health inequalities in the late twentieth century is that the NHS is not meeting its original objectives of providing free, quality health care for all, irrespective of their ability to pay. Whitehead (1988) reviews a number of studies in the debate over whether the services offered by the NHS are equally accessible to all social groups and concludes that there is evidence to suggest that access to care is, in fact, biased in favour of the non-manual socio-economic groups in terms of access, treatment and quality of care. She also proposes a further dimension of equality in health care – equal access to care for equal need – suggesting that where ill-health is greater amongst particular groups, services should be matched to their needs: that is, that there should be a form of positive action.

The reforms introduced by the NHS and Community Care Act 1990 were not only designed to improve the efficiency and cost-effectiveness of the health service, but were also specifically intended to address issues of access, equity and quality and 'to give patients, wherever they live, better health care and greater choice of the services available' (Department of Health, 1989a). The separation of the purchasers and the providers of health care and the establishment of the commissioning mechanism has placed an explicit emphasis on identifying the health needs of the resident population in the area served by the provider unit and on meeting quality standards and targets. The introduction of *The Patient's Charter* (Department of Health, 1991a) and the publication of hospital league tables are also designed to make the NHS more effective, accessible and responsive to people's health needs. While it is too soon to evaluate the impact of these reforms on inequalities in health, they have provoked widespread fears on the part of the medical and nursing professions, as well as the general public, that the principles on which the NHS were founded are under threat and that they will result in more, rather than less, inequality in health care.

But how is it possible that the NHS itself might actually contribute to the persistence of inequalities in health rather than to their reduction?

ACTIVITY 10   ALLOW **15** MINUTES

Read *Resource 3*, *'Who cares about equity in the NHS?'* (Whitehead, 1994) and then note down any ways in which the NHS might fail to provide equality in health care, thereby perpetuating inequalities in health.

Commentary

You may feel that the NHS, provided as it is on the basis of need and not ability to pay, should benefit all its users equally, depending of course on their health needs. However, the provision of a service that is free at the point of use does not necessarily ensure that there is equal access, that it is equally used in practice or that users receive equal quality of care. Whitehead suggests that the principle of equity that was the foundation of the NHS is, in fact, gradually being undermined by policy changes introduced during the 1980s and 1990s.

First, she argues, the principle of free treatment has been eroded by the increasing cost of prescriptions and charges for dental and ophthalmic treatment. In addition, the dearth of NHS dental facilities in some areas may serve to reduce the uptake. The percentage of adults visiting the dentist for a regular check-up, for example, was lower in 1991 than in 1985 in all socio-economic groups, except in the unskilled manual group although only 36% of people in this group had a check-up compared with 63% of people in social class I (Central Statistical Office, 1994a).

Second, the emphasis on community care that was introduced under the NHS and Community Care Act 1990 has brought a shift from a free service to a means-tested service for many people living in residential care or nursing homes. We shall return to this issue in later sessions.

Third, the changed system of funding for regional health authorities with the reduced weighting given to standardised mortality has resulted in a shift of resources from more deprived areas to more prosperous, healthier districts. It appears that despite attempts to reduce regional inequalities in health care provision, what Tudor Hart (1971, cited by Townsend and Davidson, 1988) termed 'the inverse care law' still operates:

> 'In areas with most sickness and death, general practitioners have more work, larger lists, less hospital support and inherit more clinically ineffective traditions of consultation than in the healthiest areas; and hospital doctors shoulder heavier caseloads with less staff and equipment, more obsolete buildings and suffer recurrent crises in the availability of beds and replacement of staff. These trends can be summed up as the inverse care law: that the availability of good medical care tends to vary inversely with the need of the population served.'

Fourth, the introduction of GP fund-holding which enables some GPs to shop around for services for their patients has led to widespread criticism that the NHS is rapidly becoming a two-tier service, with some patients having faster access to higher quality care than others.

Moreover, attempts by service providers to ensure equal access to health care are not sufficient to ensure equal treatment and equal quality in health care. As Titmuss found as long ago as 1968, higher income groups know how to make best use of the NHS because they tend to have a greater awareness of the choices available to them, to be more articulate in their demands of the service and to receive more specialist attention. Pendleton and Bochner (1980), for example, found that general practitioners commonly volunteer more explanations to middle-class patients than to those from lower social groups. People from ethnic minority communities are also often disadvantaged in their use of the NHS. Service providers have gradually recognised the importance of meeting the information needs of service users, producing different language versions of information leaflets and signposts or providing interpreting services and link workers for patients whose knowledge of English is limited. However, as Marr and Khadim (1994) show from their work with elderly Asian patients, they often fail to respond positively to the socio-cultural needs of patients and clients. In recognising the covert racism that exists in many NHS units, the Commission for Racial Equality (1994) has found it necessary to produce a race relations code of practice for maternity services to eliminate discrimination and promote equal opportunities.

There also appear to be differences in the way in which people use the NHS, with higher social groups having greater knowledge of preventive services and tending to make greater use of them. Marsh and Channing (1986), for example, conducted a study of 'deprived' patients in a GP practice, with a control group of patients from higher social groups. They found that there were 60% more hospital admissions, 75% more attendances at accident and emergency departments and nearly three times the incidence of mental illness among the sample from the lower socio-economic groups. However, they also found much lower immunisation rates, attendance at well-women and well-men clinics and uptake of other preventive services such as cervical screening among the sample compared with the control group.

More recently, Reading *et al.* (1994) have challenged the common view that improving the overall uptake of any preventive activity will also tend to reduce social inequalities in the use of preventive services because groups with the poorest uptake are likely to improve the most. In their study of an immunisation programme in the Northern Regional Health Authority, they found that despite a substantial increase in immunisation uptake, inequalities between deprived and affluent areas persisted or became wider and that any reduction in inequality only occurred after the uptake in affluent areas approached 95%. They concluded that 'improvements in the delivery of services that are applied indiscriminately across the population may leave inequalities in uptake unchanged or actually widen them because poorer members of society have less opportunity to take advantage of available services.'

For many people, opportunities to make use of services are affected by practical constraints on access. Some patients, for example, have physical difficulty in reaching health care services, particularly where they have to rely on public transport or live in rural areas. For others, the time and costs involved in actually getting to the GP's surgery or hospital clinic may be prohibitive and their attendance may be dependent on the availability of a hospital car service, subsidised public transport or help with hospital travel costs. In some areas, the problem has been exacerbated by the major reorganisation of services since the NHS reforms in 1990 with the closure of many hospital wards, accident and emergency departments and small cottage hospitals with the result that people often have further to travel for treatment. The difficulties faced by service users in reaching services may also be a significant factor in determining the use of services such as antenatal classes or child health clinics by working-class women. Dowling (1983, cited by Kendall and McAnulty, 1990) quotes one mother whose experience provides a graphic reminder that the availability of services is, in itself, insufficient to ensure equal use:

> 'You know what going to the clinic means? Three kids to get dressed and cleaned up, 25 minutes waiting for the bus – usually in the pouring rain. And then after all that, just a row of hard benches, hours and hours of waiting and those grim yellow walls. Not a toy in sight, let alone a cup of tea. God, I dread going to the clinic.'

The issue of equality in health care is, however, only one side of the coin in terms of explaining why some social groups experience poorer health than others. As

Dingwall (1979) has observed, 'comprehensive health care may make treatment equally available to all individuals but it can do nothing to ensure that the need for health care is equalised.' To understand the reasons for the persistence of inequalities in health, we need to consider some further possible explanations:

- the artefact explanation

- natural and social selection

- cultural and behavioural factors

- materialist and structural factors.

The artefact explanation

The 'artefact' explanation emphasises the difficulty, in statistical terms, of making comparisons between social classes over time. Whitehead (1988) identifies five main obstacles that need to be borne in mind in assessing research:

- numerator/denominator bias

- the reclassification of occupations at each census since 1931

- changes in the proportion of the population in each social class over time

- changes in the relative status of each social class over time

- the use of a small proportion of total deaths as a basis for comparison.

In her review of research on inequalities in health, Whitehead points to a number of studies that have attempted to overcome these obstacles and observes that their findings still indicate significant health differentials between social classes. She concludes that while it is important to be aware of the way these factors can shape the interpretation of statistical data, they do not provide a sufficient explanation for inequalities in health.

Natural and social selection

Theories of natural and social selection acknowledge the existence of social inequalities in health, but attribute them to a process of health selection. According to this explanation, people in poor health tend to move down the scale of social class and concentrate in the lower socio-economic groups, while people in good health are more likely to experience upward social mobility. A healthy worker, for example, is able to work more efficiently than one who is unhealthy and is therefore more likely to achieve greater career progression. Illsley (1986) even found that tall women are more likely to marry into a higher occupational group (height being a broad indicator of health). The gap between the higher and lower social classes therefore increases over time.

There appears, however, to be very little evidence to support explanations for health inequalities that are based on theories of health selection. While selection may account for a tiny percentage of existing health inequalities, it is generally recognised that it is social circumstances that determine health and not health that determines social position.

Cultural and behavioural factors

Cultural and behavioural explanations for inequalities in health emphasise the importance of differences in social circumstances and in the ways in which individuals in different social groups choose to lead their lives: in other words, in the behaviour and voluntary lifestyles they adopt. Thus, 'inequalities in health evolve because lower social groups have adopted more dangerous and health-damaging behaviour than the higher social groups, and may have less interest in protecting their health for the future' (Whitehead, 1988).

The cultural/behavioural explanation focuses on people's individual responsibility for their own health and the degree to which they jeopardise or enhance their chances of good health through the choices that they make about their lives. Evidence from studies such as the *General Household Survey* (1993a) and the *Health Survey for England 1991* (1993b) conducted by the Office of Population Censuses and Surveys (OPCS) shows that people in lower social groups tend to lead more unhealthy lives because they smoke more, eat less healthy food and exercise less. In 1990, for example, 16% of professional men and women smoked compared with 48% of men and 36% of women in social class V (Central Statistical Office, 1993a). However, cultural and behavioural factors are still insufficient as a full explanation of health inequalities. As Marmot *et al.* (1984) have shown, when a comparison is made between individuals from socio-economic groups I and V whose smoking, eating, drinking and exercise habits are broadly similar, health inequalities still persist.

Material and structural factors

Materialist and structuralist explanations place a greater emphasis on the external environment and the conditions under which people live and work. The importance of material deprivation as an explanation for inequalities in health is indicated by a number of studies such as that conducted for the Northern Regional Health Authority by Townsend, Phillimore and Beattie (1988) which demonstrated the deleterious effects of poor housing, unemployment, low income, inadequate facilities and services, and air pollution on health. Materialist explanations also stress the importance of socio-economic pressures on low-income households to consume unhealthy products. Graham (1984) found that when money is in short supply, spending on foods tends to be restricted and given that cheaper, but filling foods tend to be higher in sugar and fat content, this leads to less healthy diets being adopted. The widespread use of bed and breakfast accommodation to house lone parents and other homeless families, for example, has forced many families into a dependence on take-away food since much of this type of accommodation lacks cooking and refrigeration facilities.

Both the Black Report and *The Health Divide* found housing conditions to be a major contributory factor in determining health, citing data showing that people from areas of poor quality housing were in poorer health, had more long-standing illness and more symptoms of depression than those living in 'good' housing areas. As we saw in Session One, damp and mouldy housing is a major cause of respiratory and bronchial problems, while overcrowding can lead to stress within families and is a significant contributor to family breakdown and mental illness. In addition, a lack of decent amenities such as local shops, play areas for children, the poor design of inter-connecting walkways in flats, inadequate refuse collection facilities and increasing problems of infestation with their associated health risks also contribute to ill-health and accidents, especially among children (Whitehead, 1988; Young, 1980).

Employment status and unemployment have also been found to be a cause of physical and mental ill-health. Manual workers such as miners, builders and others whose jobs involve exposure to dust or toxic substances and possible accidents are clearly at greater risk of ill-health, even death, than those in professional classes. A number of studies have also shown, however, that the stress caused by unemployment is an important factor in relation to both mental and physical health. The longitudinal study undertaken by Fox and Leon (1985) demonstrated quite clearly the relationship between unemployment and health, with unemployed people experiencing a 20–30% increase in mortality, with particular increases in suicide rates, cancers and cardiovascular disease. It also showed how unemployment has a similar effect on the spouses and families of unemployed people. Further evidence of the impact of unemployment on health is to be found in studies which show that once unemployed people find their way back into work, their overall health tends to improve markedly. More recently, work by Morris *et al.* (1994) showed that apparently healthy men were twice as likely to die within 5.5 years following unemployment than men who remained continuously employed. Although they found no evidence to suggest that the relative risk associated with the loss of stable employment was any different for manual and non-manual workers, they found that the men who experienced unemployment were more likely to be manual workers and to come from the north. They also found that they were more likely to be current smokers, heavy drinkers, obese and to have reported at least two doctor diagnoses. However, adjustment for these variables suggested that neither health-related behaviour nor social factors could adequately explain the differences in mortality between the unemployed and employed men whom they studied.

For those who advance materialist and structural explanations for inequalities in health, poverty is clearly the underlying causative factor. Phillimore, Beattie and Townsend (1994), for example, found in their ongoing study in the northern region of England that mortality differentials had widened between the most affluent and deprived wards in all age categories under 75 years in 1981–91, a period of overall increase in average incomes. The decline in the relative position of the poorest areas was particularly great and there was no narrowing of inequalities across the remainder of the socio-economic spectrum. There were improvements in mortality in all age categories in the most affluent areas. In the poorest areas, however, improvements in the 55–64 age group were balanced by increased mortality among men aged 15–44, a slight rise among women aged 65–74 and static rates among men aged 45–54. They argue strongly that their study re-emphasises the case for linking mortality patterns with material conditions rather than individual behaviour:

> 'If health differentials reflected behavioural choices by individuals then worsening health would be an indication of increasingly unwise personal behaviour. Yet if historical improvements in health throughout the population are generally attributed to rising living standards and improving material conditions, so worsening health among some groups and widening differentials must be related primarily to changes in the same factors.'

A single explanation?

There remains considerable debate about the relative weight that can be attributed to behavioural and materialist factors as explanations for inequalities in health. In practice, the explanations – and therefore the policy responses that are considered appropriate – tend to be influenced by wider political perspectives. As Whitehead (1988) observes, for example, the higher incidence of childhood accidents amongst children from lower social groups could be explained by the behavioural view as being due to more reckless, risk-taking behaviour in this group and inadequate care by parents. The materialist view, however, would link the behaviour of parents and children to structural issues such as unsafe play areas, the lack of fenced-off gardens and the difficulties in supervising children in high-rise housing.

If we focus on smoking, which is a key target in the government's strategy to improve the health of the nation, we find links between behavioural and materialist factors that illustrate the difficulty of identifying clear explanations for inequalities in health. Although there has been a downward trend in smoking in recent years, it has been most marked among the better-off and scarcely evident at all in the lowest income groups. It could be argued that smoking can be seen in purely behavioural terms: a person chooses to smoke or not to smoke. Yet, as Marsh and McKay (1994) found in a re-analysis of data from the General Household Survey, the stark differential in smoking behaviour between different social groups is a recent phenomenon that directly reflects patterns of disadvantage. Their study showed that any two of a number of factors seemed to trigger a striking increase in people's likelihood to smoke, including lone parenthood, poor education, manual work, receipt of means-tested benefits and occupation of rented property. They found, for example, that the combination of low educational achievement and being a tenant seemed to lead directly to smoker status: 'What appears to have happened is that the concentration of unqualified school-leavers in the council estates of the 1970s became a protected social habitat for high levels of smoking not seen elsewhere since the early 1960s.'

Marsh and McKay also found that annual increases in the cost of cigarettes above inflation rates, the main plank of the government's anti-smoking policy, is actually contributing to increased hardship among low-income households because they are devoting a larger proportion of their disposable income to smoking. In seeking to explain why so many people cling to their habit, even though they are aware of the health hazards and both they and their children may have to go without other necessities in order to pay for it, Marsh and McKay highlight the intense stresses experienced by people in low-income groups. For the 62% of lone parents in the poorest quarter of the population who smoke, as well as many others coping with poverty, smoking is the only form of luxury they have. As they conclude, it is:

> '... the sole anodyne for family life on benefit incomes ... All modern research on how people give up smoking shows that they do so for reasons connected with optimism. Britain's lowest income parents are not people with great cause for optimism, or for self-esteem.'

The difficulty in isolating factors that provide an adequate explanation for inequalities in health is further illustrated by the Whitehall Study (Marmot *et al.*, 1984; 1986) in which health inequalities among men in different grades of the Civil Service have been examined over a period of twenty years and where the mortality rate of those in the lowest grade has been found to be three times higher than that of those in the highest grade. A similar study of the British Army by Lynch and Oelman (1981) found that the mortality rate amongst lowest-ranking members was six times higher than that amongst the highest-ranking members. Marmot *et al.* argue, however, that evidence of this kind suggests that poverty itself is an insufficient explanation for the persistence of health inequalities since, whilst the lower-grade civil servants in their study had less disposable income, they were not 'poor' as such. In addition, although lower-grade civil servants were more likely to smoke or take inadequate exercise, lifestyle factors alone did not account for the social class gradient that they found. They look instead towards an explanation that highlights psycho-social stress as an important contributor to health inequalities between different groups, an explanation that may be particularly significant when we consider the relationship between material deprivation and stress.

Their findings are strongly supported by the work on families and children by Wilkinson (1994) who has explored the relationship between income, life expectancy and the incidence of other family problems for over twenty years. His key message is that standards of health in developed countries are powerfully affected by how equal or unequal people's incomes are and that countries with the longest life expectancy are not the richest countries, but those with the smallest spread of incomes. In Britain, while average income increased by 36% between 1979 and 1990, life expectancies for men and women in the prime of life (aged 15–44) began to fall in the mid-1980s. Wilkinson found that this reflected the dramatic widening in income differences from 1985 onwards that resulted from tax and benefit changes, and changes in the structure of economic activity with rising levels of unemployment, self-employment and the number of elderly retired people. In suggesting that income inequality seems to affect health by reducing general immunity to disease, Wilkinson argues that it is not caused by the direct physiological impact of poverty, but by what people feel their circumstances to be and what the difference in their circumstances makes them feel. Thus, it is 'the social and psychological meanings attached to material differences which impact on health.' He recognises that psychological stresses are by no means confined to the poor but suggests that in increasingly unequal societies, 'the more unemployment, the more homelessness, the more houses repossessed, the more poverty, the greater will be the sense of anxiety and insecurity in the population at large.' Meanwhile, if job opportunities, pension rights and health services seem to be crumbling, people feel that there is further to fall and the risks of daily life are more worrying. As Donnison (1994) comments:

'Cautious though his interpretation is, Wilkinson's report has explosive implications. It is not poverty but inequality that damages our health. That damages our long love affair with economic growth for its own sake. Growth achieved at the cost of greater inequality is damaging: it only benefits a nation if it creates a fairer, more equal, more secure society. The assertion, beloved of economists, that we have to choose between growth and justice, efficiency and equity, is a lie ... a surrender to market morality excludes and exploits increasing numbers, destroys human relationships and blights lives.'

A strategy for health

The diversity of possible explanations for inequalities in health leads inevitably to a range of perspectives on the social policy responses that are likely to be most effective in addressing their causes. The Black Report, for example, identified material deprivation as a key factor and concluded that the more equitable distribution of health services is, in itself, insufficient to achieve a substantial reduction in health inequalities in the UK.

'While the health care service can play a significant part in reducing inequalities in health, measures to reduce differences in material standards of living at work, in the home and in everyday social and community life are of even greater importance.'

As we have seen, the Report maintained that while a proper mechanism for co-ordinating health policy was required at both national and local level, the government should make the abolition of child poverty its primary goal as a means of improving the nation's health, together with improvements in housing and working conditions. Government action would thus be required across a wide range of social and economic policy areas. The Report had been commissioned by a Labour government, but the Conservatives who had come to power before it was completed were less than enthusiastic about the findings and the policy implications. In fact, the Secretary of State, Patrick Jenkin, rejected the recommendations on the grounds that:

- the Report did not provide an adequate explanation for inequalities in health

- more recent evidence contradicted its assertion that working-class people had poor access to health services

- there was no evidence that increased funding for the NHS would improve people's health.

As the *British Medical Journal* (1986) later reported:

> 'Instead of having the report properly printed and published, the government made 260 copies of the typescript available on an August bank holiday Monday and accompanied it with a foreword from the Secretary of State stating that he had no intention of responding to its detailed recommendations. Not surprisingly, this attempt at suppression made the document instantly more newsworthy, and it has since been published by Penguin and became, in the minds of many, the most important medical report since the war.'

Six years later, the *Registrar General's Decennial Supplement on Occupational Mortality* (OPCS, 1986) was published, analysing deaths by occupation, cause of death, sex and age. For the first time, no reference was made to social class differences in mortality on the grounds that changes in the classification of occupations had made some of the data unreliable, particularly those relating to social class V. As Kendall and McAnulty (1990) report, one of the authors published some of the data simultaneously elsewhere and overcame the problems resulting from the changes in classification, showing that inequalities in health between the social classes were, in fact, increasing. This prompted the *British Medical Journal* (1986) to question whether the government was suppressing potentially adverse information, asking, 'Why is this? Could it be because somebody in the government or in the Registrar General's office is anxious to play down the widening gap in mortality between rich and poor?'

Some eight years after the publication of the Black Report, concern was expressed in *The Health Divide* that none of its recommendations had been implemented.

> 'In reality what has happened over the past eight years is a disturbing increase in the number of children growing up in poverty, and an increase in families becoming homeless. Policies deliberately designed to reduce child poverty have not been adopted, and the situation has been exacerbated by a sharp rise in the level of unemployment which has affected families with young children in particular. A concerted effort to improve housing conditions has not been made and there is

now growing concern over the shortage of houses and the poor state of repair of existing dwellings ... Mechanisms for co-ordinating policies on health in local and national government have not been set up ... although it is widely acknowledged that health promotion policies need to involve many agencies outside the health sector, such as housing, environmental control, transport, food and agriculture and – above all – the Treasury.'

By the early 1990s, it was clear that government action to improve health would continue to be focused specifically on health issues rather than wider social and economic factors. As we have seen, the reorganisation of the health service following the publication of the White Paper, *Working for Patients* (Department of Health, 1989a) and the introduction of the NHS and Community Care Act 1990 was designed to produce an efficient, cost-effective service that is more responsive to patients' needs. It has been accompanied by a greater focus on preventive health care with the implementation of the strategy outlined in the government White Paper, *The Health of the Nation: A strategy for health in England* (Department of Health, 1992), and equivalent policy documents in Wales, Scotland and Northern Ireland. In the final part of this session, we shall consider the potential of this strategy to overcome some of the inequalities in health that demonstrably exist.

The Health of the Nation

The Health of the Nation strategy is a major development in public health policy because, while acknowledging that further improvement of treatment, care and rehabilitation remains essential, it marks a greater emphasis on the promotion of health and the prevention of disease. The strategy encompasses the following approaches:

- the selection of five key areas for action:
  - coronary heart disease and stroke
  - cancers
  - mental illness
  - accidents
  - HIV/AIDS and sexual health

- setting national objectives and targets in the key areas

- indicating the action needed to achieve the targets

- outlining initiatives to help implement the strategy

- setting the framework for monitoring, development and review.

The introduction of the strategy was preceded by the publication of a consultative document, *The Health of the Nation* (Department of Health, 1991b) which aimed to stimulate widespread public and professional debate on health and how it might be improved. As the Secretary of State for Health, Virginia Bottomley, commented in the foreword to the White Paper, the overall strategy attracted very wide backing:

'There was support for the need to concentrate on health promotion as much as health care; for the need to set clear and challenging targets – and not too many of them – at which to aim; and for the need for all of us to work together. These principles are essential if we are to make a further significant improvement in the health of the people.'

The White Paper acknowledged that the government is responsible for many elements vital to ensuring a healthy population, including:

- legislation and regulation

- providing reliable information on which individuals can base their decisions on matters that affect their health

- facilitating and encouraging action

- allocating resources

- monitoring and assessing changes in health.

In setting clear targets for the improvement of the nation's health, however, a balance is envisaged between the contribution of the government and the NHS, statutory and other authorities, the Health Education Authority, voluntary bodies, employers and employees and the media:

'... although there is much that Government and the NHS needs to do, the objectives and targets cannot be delivered by Government and the NHS alone. They are truly for the nation – for all of us – to achieve. We must be clear about where responsibilities lie. We must get the balance right between what the Government, and Government alone, can do, what other organisations and agencies need to do, and finally, what individuals and families themselves must contribute if the strategy is to succeed.'
(Department of Health, 1992)

In placing a firm emphasis on health education to help individuals make the right choices about health, the Department of Health stresses that the impact on health can often be greater when individuals and organisations work together. The strategy thus places high priority on the establishment of active partnerships or 'healthy alliances' in a variety of settings in which people live and work and which, between them, offer the potential to involve most people in the country:

- healthy cities

- healthy schools

- healthy hospitals

- healthy workplaces

- healthy homes

- healthy environments.

ACTIVITY II

Read *Resource 4, 'The targets in full'* (Department of Health, 1992) which outlines the Health of the Nation targets for England and *Resource 5, 'Making the strategy work'* (Department of Health, 1992), which focuses on policy implementation and considers the role of 'healthy alliances'. Then note down your thoughts on the extent to which this major health promotion initiative might have a direct impact on inequalities in health.

Commentary

The Health of the Nation is a significant advance in the achievement of better health for all through its promotion of good health and prevention of ill-health in the five key areas which are the major causes of serious illness or early death. In its overall aim of improving the extent and effectiveness of public education – and, hence, stimulating changes in lifestyle – it specifically attempts to address cultural and behavioural factors that contribute to ill-health and, indeed, to inequalities in health. Thus, particular emphasis is placed on health education about diet, alcohol use, exercise, smoking, HIV and AIDS and safety at home and on the roads in order to promote lifestyle changes.

The strategy also aims to promote increased uptake of services such as immunisation and screening for conditions such as breast cancer and cervical cancer. Improved information and communication, coupled with incentives for GPs and other service providers to meet targets, are expected to have a tangible effect in reaching sectors of the population which have traditionally made less use of preventive services. Although the results are encouraging, Reading *et al.* (1994) cautioned in their study of interventions to improve the uptake of immunisation that any improvement or increase that is applied across a population and that results in a general improvement in health will not necessarily reduce social inequalities in health and may actually widen them.

> 'This does not mean that social inequalities in the uptake of preventive activities cannot be changed. Marsh and Channing showed that prioritising services to a deprived estate in their primary health care practice resulted in the virtual abolition of social inequalities in a range of preventive activities. The important difference between that study and ours is that their primary aim was the reduction of social inequalities in coverage rather than an improvement in overall levels of coverage. It appears that we cannot rely on a general improvement in the efficiency of a service to narrow any inequalities in uptake; we have to direct specific measures towards improving social equity in uptake as well. This in turn has resource implications. The health service and ultimately society as a whole has to decide how much of their resources should be used in improving social equity in the delivery and uptake of services.'

While the strategy focuses on health promotion and increasing the effectiveness of preventive health services, the White Paper acknowledges that many policies have, to a greater or lesser extent, an impact on health and that it is therefore important that 'as policy is developed the consequences for health are assessed and, where appropriate, taken into account.' It thus identifies one of the most important tasks for government as ensuring that government departments work together, with the establishment of a Ministerial Cabinet Committee covering eleven departments to oversee implementation, monitoring and development. Nevertheless, it is possible to identify a number of ways in which the policies of different departments fail to support the Health of the Nation strategy. The refusal of the government to ban tobacco advertising, for example, is considered by many health professionals to be a critical weakness in its attempts to reduce smoking, particularly among young people. In November 1993, a year after the introduction of the strategy, the Department of Health admitted that teenage smoking had remained static, although the target was for a reduction in smoking prevalence amongst 11–15 year olds of at least 33% by 1994 (from about 8% in 1988 to less than 6%). Department for Education guidelines placing constraints on teaching about contraception and safer sex in schools can similarly be seen as undermining the achievement of targets set by the Department of Health to reduce the rate of unplanned pregnancies among under 16-year-olds and to halt the transmission of HIV.

The White Paper makes limited reference to the ways in which the strategy will address material and structural factors contributing to ill-health and inequalities in health. It recognises the broad link between a decent local environment and housing conditions and good health, citing the role of Housing Action Trusts, Estate Action and the Urban Programme in promoting urban renewal, and City Challenge as a stimulus to local authorities to make particularly deprived areas more attractive and healthier places in which to live and work. Nevertheless, it makes no direct reference to the role of social inequality in causing illness. Thus, in the section on healthy homes, it states that good housing is important to good health, but that 'the interdependence between factors such as occupational class, income, unemployment, housing and lifestyle makes it difficult to assess which health effects are specifically attributable to it.'

Despite the undoubted importance and value of the Health of the Nation initiative, its failure to address the ways in which issues of poverty and inequality interrelate with individual lifestyle decisions is thought by many health care professionals and researchers to undermine its potential effectiveness in reducing continuing differentials in health. In May 1994, however, the government made an apparent U-turn with the announcement to a British Medical Association conference on social inequalities and health that a new sub-committee was being established to investigate the links between poverty and ill-health, as part of its continuing review of Health of the Nation targets. In a message to the conference, the Secretary of State for Health, Virginia Bottomley, said that 'The reasons for these variations are likely to be the result of a complex interplay of genetics, biological, social, environmental, cultural and behavioural factors. We need a better understanding of how these factors interrelate and at what points it is possible to undertake effective interventions.'

Some researchers into health inequalities have pointed out that a considerable body of evidence already exists on the causes of health inequalities and the most effective ways of tackling them, and that the need is for action rather than more research and discussion. Nevertheless, after years of official reluctance to acknowledge the impact of social inequalities on health, the inquiry is an indication of government recognition of the need to move towards a broader agenda in tackling the problems of ill-health.

In Session Three, we shall explore another area of social policy, community care, and consider the changing roles of the statutory, private, voluntary and informal sectors in the 'mixed economy of welfare'.

Summary

1   Improvements in health during the twentieth century have resulted from improved social, economic and environmental conditions as well as from advances in medical technology and wider access to health care through the National Health Service.

2   Despite overall improvements in health, significant inequalities in health persist in the UK, as shown by social class, regional, gender and ethnic variations in mortality and morbidity rates.

3   Policy changes in the 1980s and 1990s resulting in the reorganisation of health service funding and delivery may undermine the principles of equality that were the foundation of the National Health Service.

4   There is no single explanation for inequalities in health. Interlinking cultural/behavioural and material/structural factors may be exacerbated by psycho-social stress and constraints on the use of the NHS by poorer social groups.

5   The Health of the Nation initiative emphasises health promotion and disease prevention as much as health care as a means of achieving further improvements in health. It focuses on cultural and behavioural factors contributing to ill-health rather than on material and structural factors.

Before you move on to Session Three, check that you have achieved the objectives given at the beginning of this session and, if not, review the appropriate sections.

SESSION THREE

The mixed economy of welfare

Introduction

In this session, we shall consider the contribution of the four main sectors involved in the implementation of social policy: the statutory, private, voluntary and informal sectors. Together, they form what is known as 'the mixed economy of welfare'. In particular, we shall explore the interrelationship between these four sectors by focusing on the development of community care policies. As you will see in this session and the next four sessions, since 1979 there has been a major shift away from direct provision by the statutory sector towards the commissioning of services from both the private and voluntary sectors, as well as an increasing reliance on informal care.

Session objectives

When you have completed this session, you should be able to:

- describe the roles of the four main sectors in the mixed economy of welfare

- outline the provisions of the NHS and Community Care Act 1990

- identify the providers of community care services in your local area.

Who provides welfare services?

Throughout this unit, we place a great deal of emphasis on the interdependence of different areas of social policy and on the interaction between them. In Session Two, for instance, we considered a number of studies on health inequalities in the UK which highlight the influence of social policy areas such as housing, employment and social security and wider economic policy on health. In this session, however, we shall focus on the role of different providers of welfare within specific areas of social policy and on the interaction between these providers and the range of services that they offer.

It is important to recognise that welfare services are not provided exclusively by the statutory sector – that is, by central government and local authorities. Consider, for example, the many different providers of housing. We saw in Session One that housing is provided by:

- the statutory sector: local authority housing

- the private sector: home ownership and private renting

- the voluntary sector: housing associations

- the informal sector: parents, family or friends.

ACTIVITY 12   ALLOW 5 MINUTES

Just as housing is provided by the statutory, private, voluntary and informal sectors, so too are other areas of welfare services. Can you think of an example of another area of social policy in which services are provided by at least three of these four sectors?

Commentary

Education is an obvious example of provision by all four sectors, although data from the Central Statistical Office (1994a) show that the balance between them varies considerably according to the level at which education is being provided and that some sectors have shown considerable change over time. By 1991/92, 53% of all children aged three or four were attending school, compared with only

15% in 1965/66. While there had been a large increase in the number of under-fives attending primary school on a full-time or part-time basis, part-time attendance had increased eight-fold for nursery schools and ten-fold for non-maintained (private) schools. There had also been a seven-fold increase in the number of under-fives catered for by child-minders and in local authority, private, voluntary and workplace day nurseries and playgroups. In 1991, almost two-fifths of working mothers were using unpaid family and friends to care for their children, with those working full-time more than twice as likely to use a paid child-minder or nanny than those working part-time.

While the majority of children go to state primary and secondary schools, there has been a small expansion of the private sector, with 7% of all children attending independent schools compared with 5% in 1975/76. The percentage increases with age, however; in 1991/92, 5% of under-elevens attended independent schools compared with 18% of boys and 15% of girls aged 16 and over. Some children attend religious schools or special schools run by voluntary organisations such as SCOPE, while others are educated within the home on a full- or part-time basis by their parents. During the period 1970 and 1981, there was a large increase in the number of children in special schools when education authorities took over responsibility from the health authorities for schools catering for children with physical or learning disabilities. Since 1985/86, however, the number of children allocated a place in an ordinary public sector school rather than in a special school has more than doubled.

Further and higher education tend to be provided largely by the public sector, although the voluntary sector has traditionally played an important role in adult education through such organisations as the Workers Educational Association and trade unions. In 1992, more than three-fifths of people teaching basic literacy and numeracy skills were volunteers; the remainder were employed by local education authorities, voluntary groups, employment training schemes, colleges of further education, penal establishments and the Adult Literacy and Basic Skills Unit.

As you will see later in this session and subsequent sessions, health care and the personal social services are the other main areas in which all four sectors play a part in service provision.

The system of welfare provision in which the statutory, private, voluntary and informal sectors all provide a range of services has come to be known as the 'mixed economy of welfare'. This means that, in practice, all four of the main sectors or welfare providers have a role to play in the implementation of social policy. In contrast, welfare systems in some countries place almost sole emphasis on the government's role in meeting welfare needs, as in many of the former communist states, or on the role of the private sector in welfare provision; in the United States, for example, health care is largely provided through the private sector with employers funding health insurance for nearly 60% of the population.

In the next four sessions, we shall look in more detail at the advantages and disadvantages of the changing roles of the four main sectors as providers of social welfare. The aim of this session, however, is to introduce you to these sectors and to encourage you to recognise the interaction that takes place between them.

The statutory sector and the role of the state

The statutory sector includes public authorities or bodies that have been created by law and are largely paid for through taxation. These include the Benefits Agency, social services departments, health authorities, local education authorities and housing departments. Although direct service provision is the most obvious function of the statutory sector, it has a wider role in commissioning, financing, regulating and coordinating services that are provided by other sectors.

Service provision

Some services are provided by central government and local authorities on a mandatory basis; in other words, they have a duty under law to provide them. These services include education for children between the ages of 5–16, hospital and community health services, social security benefits, state retirement pensions and the provision of some form of housing for the involuntary homeless.

Other services are provided on a discretionary basis; that is, government and local authorities have the power to provide them, but are not obliged to do so because there is no legal requirement to offer them. These services include recreation and leisure services, pre-school education, day centres and home care assistants for elderly people and people with physical or learning disabilities, meals-on-wheels services and concessionary travel passes for elderly people.

Funding

In addition to its function of direct service provision, the state's involvement in the provision of welfare includes the financing of services provided by the private, voluntary or informal sectors. Since 1979, the rapid expansion of private sector provision has been promoted by the use of public funds to pay for welfare services and, increasingly, local authorities and health authorities are commissioning private suppliers to provide the services they decide are needed in their areas.

Many voluntary organisations such as the National Association of Citizens Advice Bureaux (NACAB) and Barnardo's have long received grants from central or local government but, like the private sector, they are increasingly being contracted to provide services. In the informal sector, many family carers receive an invalid care allowance.

Regulation

The state also has an important regulatory role in welfare provision through standard setting, monitoring and inspection. Charities, for instance, are regulated by legislation which requires them to satisfy the requirements of the Charity Commissioners, while schools and many welfare services provided by the voluntary and private sectors are subject to inspection in order to ensure that they meet specified standards. Under the Registered Homes Act 1984, local authority, private and voluntary residential care homes are registered and inspected by local authorities and nursing homes are inspected by health authorities. With the shift to the commissioning of services by the state, clear specifications relating to cost and quality are set in service contracts which must be met by those providing the services, whether statutory, private or voluntary sector providers.

Co-ordination

The fourth role of the state is to co-ordinate the planning and delivery of welfare services in order to ensure that they meet the needs of service users and to avoid gaps or duplication in services. Under the NHS and Community Care Act 1990, for example, local authorities were designated as the 'lead authority' in service planning and were required to prepare and publish community care plans in consultation with district health authorities and family health services authorities, voluntary housing agencies and voluntary organisations representing service users or their carers. The government subsequently issued a directive also requiring them to consult with local independent suppliers in the planning of services. Local authorities therefore play a key role in ensuring that the different agencies involved work together effectively in the provision of community care.

The private sector

The private or independent sector consists of companies, organisations or individuals that sell their services in order to make a profit and ranges from large corporations, such as companies building or providing retirement housing to small domestic care agencies. The charges for their services may be paid directly by the recipients but may also be paid by the state which commissions or contracts them to provide those services on its behalf. Under the 1990 NHS reforms, for example, the purchasers of health care, whether purchasing commissions in health authorities or GP fundholders, are free to commission services from private hospitals and community services as well as from NHS providers. In the area of community care, special rates of supplementary benefit and, later, income support were paid to people in private residential and nursing homes who were deemed eligible by a financial means test. In April 1993, a new funding structure was introduced and social services departments took responsibility for the financial support of people in private and voluntary homes, with the level of the individual's contribution to the fees being determined by their capital and income, including social security benefits.

There are also other, less obvious, examples of the interaction between the statutory and private sectors, such as indirect state support through tax concessions to employers for private health insurance schemes, tax relief on private pensions and mortgage interest tax relief for individual home-owners.

The voluntary sector

The voluntary sector consists of charities and non-profit-making voluntary organisations which provide services or represent particular groups or interests. They range from large national organisations with local branches, such as Age Concern, the National Association for Mental Health (MIND) and the Pre-School Playgroups Association to small local organisations such as self-help networks, voluntary hospices or pensioners' associations. Many provide specialised services through paid staff or trained volunteers or help to co-ordinate and support the activities of local groups concerned with the welfare of specific client groups. Some, including many self-advocacy groups, focus particularly on education and campaigning. The voluntary sector also includes housing associations, many of whom specialise in provision for people with particular needs, such as elderly people or young single homeless people.

Voluntary organisations receive funding from a variety of sources. Some are dependent on charitable donations from individuals and companies, corporate sponsorship and their charity shops and other business activities to finance the services they provide. Over 90% of the NSPCC's income, for example, comes from the public. However, voluntary organisations often rely heavily on funding from central and local government, without which many would be unable to provide services. Traditionally, many voluntary organisations have received grants from local authorities to support their work which are not necessarily tied to a particular service or activity. Increasingly, however, services are being commissioned by local authorities, particularly where long-term funding or substantial payments are involved. It is important to recognise the extent to which many voluntary organisations rely on state funding as it illustrates the financing role of the state in the mixed economy of welfare and the degree of interdependency which exists between the sectors and the services they provide.

The informal sector

The term 'informal sector' is commonly used to describe a wide range of services provided for dependent people in their own homes on an unpaid basis by family and friends. These range from assisting with personal care activities, such as washing and toileting, through general household duties to providing emotional and social support and keeping an eye on vulnerable people. We shall explore these services in more detail in Session Seven. Many of these tasks may not seem to be unduly demanding and, for those carrying them out for a loved one, may not normally be thought of as work. Nevertheless, they are essential tasks that have to be undertaken if people who are dependent are to remain within their own homes or in the community. If they are not performed by carers, they have to be carried out by one of the other sectors: by district nurses, home care assistants, social workers, the meals-on-wheels service, residential care workers, wardens in sheltered accommodation, and so on.

Community care

In order to analyse some of the ways in which the four sectors interact with one another, both within and between different areas of social policy, we shall now focus more specifically on the area of community care. Community care is used as an example here because it represents a central plank of government social policy for the 1990s and it is an area of social welfare in which each sector plays an important role.

Meredith (1993) defines community care in broad terms as 'helping people who need care and support to live with dignity and as much independence as possible "in the community".' The primary aim is to provide a range of services to enable people who have care needs to remain integrated within the community and not separate from it so that they can, as far as possible, maintain an independent way of life. Ideally, this means enabling them to remain within their own homes or those of their families. If these options are not available or viable, the preferred alternative is for them to move into small residential care or nursing homes within the community rather than into long-stay hospitals or large, often isolated, residential institutions which community care seeks to replace. Community care is not simply an alternative to institutional care because it is designed to provide a continuum of support including domiciliary, day, residential, nursing and respite care services for a number of adult and child client groups, including:

- elderly people
- people with physical disabilities
- people with learning disabilities
- people with mental health problems
- people with drug or alcohol problems
- people with HIV or AIDS
- people who are terminally ill.

What kind of care do you think might be needed by people who cannot manage on their own without support in order to continue living within the community?

ACTIVITY 13

In order to appreciate the range of services that have to be made available by providers of community care, make a list of some of the difficulties and care needs that you think elderly people living alone might encounter. What services might be required to enable them to remain living in their own homes and maintain, as much as possible, a 'normal' way of life? You may find it helpful to think of an elderly person whom you know, either personally or professionally.

Commentary

While the needs of elderly people obviously vary widely, your answers are likely to fall into the following broad areas:

Financial support

Many elderly people live on very low incomes. The Central Statistical Office (1994b) reports that, in 1993, pensioners were dependent on social security benefits for 48% of their household income, in contrast to 13.9% for the average household. This means that many experience difficulties in meeting the costs of rent or the maintenance of owner-occupied property, council tax, high heating costs, transportation, a television licence and healthy food.

While many elderly people receive occupational or private pensions in addition to state retirement pensions and war pensions, many face difficulties in providing for their own needs. The financial problems that they may experience can be alleviated by benefits such as income support, housing benefit, council tax benefit, attendance allowance, heating allowances and exemption from VAT on fuel, free prescriptions and financial help from family or friends. Many elderly people are also entitled to free sight tests and vouchers for glasses, dental treatment and hearing aids.

Health and social care

By no means all elderly people suffer from ill-health but, as a group, they are more likely to suffer from chronic diseases such as arthritis or degenerative diseases such as dementias. Many of the health problems typically associated with elderly people not only require frequent medical or nursing attention, but may also reduce personal mobility or the capacity for self-care. As a result, they may be housebound, dependent on a wheelchair or unable to manage stairs easily. They may be unable to cook their own meals, keep the house clean and tidy, wash and dress themselves or administer their own medication.

Health and social care needs are met by a range of service providers, including social workers who are responsible for assessing individuals' needs, general practitioners, district nurses, community psychiatric nurses and home care assistants, as well as family, neighbours and friends who may help with personal hygiene, cooking and cleaning. Other support may be provided by meals-on-wheels services and occupational therapists who assess the need for aids and equipment such as rails, wheelchairs, ramps and stairlifts in order to improve safety and mobility within the home. Sheltered housing may be available through the local authority, a voluntary organisation or the private sector.

Emotional support and social interaction

Many elderly people suffer from isolation either because they have no family or friends, or because they live some distance away from them. As a result, their opportunities for social interaction and emotional support may be extremely limited. Even where family and friends are within visiting distance, elderly people are often unable to leave their homes because of limited mobility or inadequate public transport or are reluctant to do so for fear of crime.

Many social problems can be overcome by access to day care centres and luncheon clubs which provide opportunities for interaction with others. The availability of free or subsidised transport, outings and cheap cinema tickets enable elderly people to participate in community life and take advantage of local recreation and leisure facilities, while home visits by family, friends and volunteers meet a range of emotional and practical support needs.

Whilst this list is by no means exhaustive, it does illustrate the range of services required to meet the aims of community care in alleviating some of the problems faced by many elderly people living alone in their own homes. Having looked at some of the services which are provided as part of community care programmes, let us consider the way in which the mixed economy of welfare now operates to provide those services.

The mixed economy of welfare in action: the community care reforms

As we have seen, the functions of funding, regulation and co-ordination have always been important components of the role of the statutory sector. Nevertheless, most public health and social services are planned and provided by the statutory sector and this has remained its principal function. Since 1979, however, there has been a clear policy shift, particularly in the areas of housing, health and social services, with a change in the role of the statutory sector from a direct service provision role to an 'enabling' role which, it is said by the Conservative government, will:

- offer more choice of services

- provide services that meet individual needs in a more flexible and innovative way

- encourage competition between providers in order to achieve more efficient and cost-effective service provision.

As a consequence, greater emphasis is now being placed on the roles of the private, voluntary and informal sectors in the mixed economy of welfare. Nowhere is this more evident than in the recent changes in community care policy and practice.

As Meredith (1993) reminds us, community care has been around for many years and it is important not to equate it with the community care changes introduced in April 1993 under the provisions of the NHS and Community Care Act. She suggests that the ideal of community care is widely supported because of a common belief that:

- people would rather be cared for in their own homes or in small home-like institutions

- it is better to care for people outside large institutions which cannot offer personalised, stimulating environments for either residents or staff

- it is important to value the worth and dignity of each person needing care

- the reorganisation of services, authorities and professional ways of working will improve services.

In exploring the reasons for the major changes that have been introduced in community care, she also points to a number of concerns about its practice, which has varied in quality and coverage and has often been found to be deficient, as well as the influence of philosophies and ideologies that have shaped social policy since the Conservatives came to power in 1979. These include:

- a concern with the high cost of care in institutions and a belief that care at home is cheaper

- an inability of different authorities and organisations to work constructively together to improve services

- the struggle to give priority to the care of people with chronic illness or disabling conditions

- competition between client groups when resources are stretched

- a conflict between the belief that services are most appropriately planned and provided at local level with the need, as seen by successive governments, to reduce or tightly control public expenditure

- a gradual change in the philosophy of public services from universal provision, available as of right and according to need, to selective provision, dependent on means and limited to those in greatest need

- a change in the philosophy of public social provision to a mixed economy, with more emphasis on the private and voluntary sectors as providers

- a move from support for collective – or state – provision to a belief that individuals should take increasing responsibility for themselves.

The introduction of the community care reforms under the NHS and Community Care Act 1990 exemplifies the commitment of the Conservative government to focus services more directly on meeting the needs of service users while limiting public expenditure. They aim to achieve this by targeting services on those in greatest need and by separating the purchasers and providers of services in order to introduce market forces and encourage a mixed economy of welfare, with an emphasis on private, voluntary and informal care services rather than public sector provision.

The roots of the community care changes lie in two key reports. In 1986, the Audit Commission published *Making a Reality of Community Care*, which suggested that the availability of supplementary benefit payments for residential and nursing home care were 'skewing' public expenditure for people with care needs. As Meredith observes, it was seen to be too easy for people to go into homes with public support and this was discouraging the development of effective services for people in their own homes. Subsequently, the government requested Sir Roy Griffiths to look at the organisation and funding of community care services. His influential report, *Community Care: An Agenda for action* (1988), formed the basis for the changes that were outlined in the White Paper, *Caring for People* (Department of Health, 1989b). The required legal changes were set out in the NHS and Community Care Act 1990 and in April 1993, the new procedures for arranging and paying for state-funded social care came into force.

The six key objectives set out in *Caring for People* indicate a clear change in the balance envisaged between the different sectors in the mixed economy of welfare and the shift to an enabling role on the part of the statutory sector.

'1 To promote the development of domiciliary, day and respite services to enable people to live in their own homes wherever feasible and sensible... in future, the Government will encourage the targeting of home-based services on those people whose need for them is greatest.

2 To ensure that service providers make practical support for carers a high priority.

3 To make proper assessment of need and good case management the cornerstone of high quality care. Packages of care should then be designed in line with individual needs and preferences.

4 To promote the development of a flourishing independent sector alongside good quality public services ... social services authorities should be "enabling" agencies. It will be their responsibility to make maximum possible use of private and voluntary providers.

5 To clarify the responsibilities of agencies and so make it easier to hold them to account for their performance.

6 To secure better value for taxpayers' money by introducing a new funding structure for social care ... social security provision should not ... provide any incentive in favour of residential and nursing home care.'

The White Paper provided for special social security allowances for residential and nursing home care to be abolished, with the money that this would cost being given to local authorities to make arrangements for care. In addition, the role of local authority social services departments has explicitly shifted from direct service provision to the 'enabling' function recommended in the Griffiths Report. As the Department of Health Social Services Inspectorate's Practice Guidance (1991) on purchasing and contracting states, the role of the local authority is:

'to identify the needs for care among the population it serves, plan how best to meet those needs, set overall strategies, priorities and targets, commission and purchase, as well as provide necessary services and ensure their quality and value.'

Social services departments have been made responsible, in collaboration with medical, nursing and other interests, for assessing individual need, designing care arrangements and securing their delivery within available resources. They are expected to produce and publish clear plans for the development of community care services, consistent with the plans of health authorities and other interested agencies and to show that they are making maximum use of the independent sector. As *Caring for People* explicitly stated:

'The Government will expect local authorities to make use wherever possible of services from voluntary, 'not for profit' and private providers insofar as this represents a cost-effective care choice. Social services authorities will continue to play a valuable role in the provision of services, but in those cases where they are still the main or sole providers of services, they will be expected to take all steps to secure diversity of provision ... [they] will be expected to make clear in their community care plans what steps they will be taking to make increased use of non-statutory service providers or, where such providers are not currently available, how they propose to stimulate such activity.'

Indeed, in the first year of the funding transfer, local authorities were required to spend at least 85% of the 'transfer element' of the Special Transitional Grant in the voluntary and private sectors through such activities as:

- devising specifications of service requirements and arrangements for tenders and contracts

- stimulating the establishment of 'not for profit' agencies

- identifying self-contained areas of their own work that could be floated off as self-managing units

- stimulating the development of new voluntary sector activity.

Caring for People also confirmed the central role of carers as providers of community care, in line with the proposals contained in the Griffiths Report (1988) which had stated that:

'Publicly provided services constitute only a small part of the total care provided to people in need. Families, friends, neighbours and other local people provide the majority of care in response to needs which they are uniquely well placed to identify and respond to. This will be the primary means by which people are enabled to live normal lives in community settings ... The proposals take as their starting point that this is as it should be and that the first task of publicly provided services is to support and, where possible, strengthen these networks of carers. Public services can help by identifying such actual and potential carers, consulting them about their needs and those of the people they are caring for and tailoring the provision of extra services (if required) accordingly.'

As Becker *et al.* (1993) observe, having established that the prime responsibility for community care should rest with local authorities, the Griffiths Report (1988) highlighted what relatively minor players the statutory services would actually be in the overall provision of care.

The provision of services

In order to see how the interaction between the statutory, private, voluntary and informal sectors operates, we shall focus on some brief case studies that illustrate:

- some of the needs experienced by individuals who are unable to live independently

- the services that may be provided to meet these needs

- the respective roles of the different sectors in service provision.

ACTIVITY 14   ALLOW **10** MINUTES

Read through the three case studies which follow. Note down in the empty brackets the sector that provides the services which each person receives.

Trevor

Trevor is 23 and has learning difficulties. He is physically disabled and confined to a wheelchair as a result of cerebral palsy.

A Trevor lives with his retired parents in their two-storey house. [   ]

B Trevor's parents are applying for a grant from the local authority to convert part of the ground floor into a bathroom and bedroom for him. [   ]

C Trevor receives a disability living allowance and his parents receive income support. [   ]

D Following assessment by his social worker [   ] the local authority has recently arranged for Trevor to attend a resource and activity centre run by a new independent organisation on two days a week. [   ] Once a week he goes to a Gateway club run by a local voluntary organisation. [   ]

E Trevor receives physiotherapy at the local hospital. [   ]

F He uses an electric wheelchair which his parents bought and maintain. [   ]

G He recently had an operation on the NHS to prevent stiffening of his legs. [   ]

John

John is 30 and was diagnosed as being HIV positive five years ago. He developed full-blown AIDS two years ago.

A John lives in his own home and is cared for by his partner who works full-time [   ] with help from a home care assistant. [   ]

B John's partner is finding it increasingly difficult to cope with his deteriorating condition. As a result, there are plans to move him into a hospice. [   ]

C Throughout his illness, John and his partner have received counselling through a service run by the Terrence Higgins Trust [   ] which has helped them come to terms with some of the difficulties they face and has also put them in touch with others in similar circumstances.

D John also receives practical and emotional support through the 'buddy' service operated by the Terrence Higgins Trust. [   ]

E John receives regular visits from the district nurse and GP and has recently spent a period of two weeks in hospital after developing pneumonia. [   ]

F John receives a disability living allowance. [   ]

Mary and Jack

Jack is 74. Mary, his wife, died recently at the age of 71.

A In the last five years of her life, Mary had become increasingly dependent on her husband to look after her because of her arthritis. [   ]

B In the year before she died, Mary's memory and behaviour deteriorated rapidly and she was diagnosed by their GP as suffering from senile dementia. [   ]

C Following the diagnosis, a social worker assessed Mary and Jack's needs. [   ] As a result, Mary went into the local hospital for a short period of respite care where, after assessment, she was treated for her condition and given occupational therapy and physiotherapy. [   ]

D It was decided that it was in Mary's best interests for her to move into a private residential care home catering for people with dementia. [   ] Part of the fees for the residential home were met by the social services department [   ] but Mary and Jack had to make a substantial contribution to the cost from their savings and pensions. [   ]

E After Mary died, Jack left the sheltered housing run by a local housing association [   ] in which he and Mary had lived and went to live with their daughter. [   ]

F Jack receives a small occupational pension [   ] as well as the state retirement pension. [   ]

G During the day, Jack often visits the local cinema as it is cheaper for pensioners in the afternoons. [   ] He uses his pensioners' travel pass on the local bus service to get there. [   ]

H On Wednesdays, Jack visits a day centre for elderly people run by a local voluntary group. [   ] However, the local authority has recently withdrawn its funding for the centre and it may have to close down. [   ]

Commentary

You probably found it easy to identify the different sectors involved in the provision of services which illustrate the way in which the mixed economy of welfare operates.

Trevor

A: informal. B: statutory. C: statutory. D: statutory; private, with statutory funding; voluntary. E: statutory. F: private. G: statutory.

John

A: informal; statutory. B: usually voluntary. C: voluntary. D: voluntary. E: statutory. F: statutory.

Mary and Jack

A: informal. B: statutory. C: statutory. D: private; statutory; informal. E: voluntary; informal. F: private; statutory. G: private; statutory. H: voluntary; statutory funding.

How familiar are you with the variety of services that are available in your own area? *Offprint 6*, an excerpt from *Take Care*, a Radio 4 factsheet, outlines local sources of information about community care services.

ACTIVITY 15   ALLOW **90 MINUTES**

Read *Resource 6, Getting the social and health care you need* (BBC, 1991). Then, using the suggestions for sources of information given in the factsheet or by talking to some people who receive community care services, find out the services available in your own area that might help to meet the needs of an elderly person such as Sarah. You may prefer to focus on someone you know, perhaps the person whose needs you identified in *Activity 13*.

Sarah

Sarah is 74 and lives alone in her small council house. She has no savings and relies on her state pension. Although she has no family, her neighbour is friendly and visits her regularly. Sarah is quite frail and her mobility is severely restricted. This makes it difficult for her to wash, dress, cook and keep her home clean and tidy. Because of her limited mobility, Sarah is rarely able to get out of her house to collect her pension, go shopping or meet other people. Her home is also in need of some internal repair. Sarah's GP has suggested that it might be better for her to move into a small residential care home.

Commentary

In order to find out about services available in your area, you will need to have considered the following questions:

- Where could Sarah get advice on whether she is entitled to additional benefits such as income support, housing benefit and council tax benefit?

- Who provides home helps and meals-on-wheels? Is there a charge for these services? If so, how much?

- What aids, adaptations or equipment could be provided to improve Sarah's mobility?

- Is there a local voluntary agency that arranges for elderly people to be visited in their own homes?

- What services, such as day centres or luncheon clubs, are available to help overcome Sarah's social isolation?

- Are there any free or subsidised transportation services that Sarah could use to attend them?

- Does your local cinema give discounts for elderly people?

- Are there any agency services, such as Care and Repair or Staying Put, that could help to adapt or improve Sarah's home?

- What residential care homes are there in your local area? Are they run by the private sector, the statutory sector or the voluntary sector? How much do they cost?

- Are there any sheltered housing schemes? Which sector provides them in your area?

As the factsheet indicates, the first port of call for Sarah should be the local social services department which is responsible for assessing her needs, providing information and making arrangements for any services she may require under community care legislation, including admission to a residential care home. If she decides to remain in her own home, the social worker should help her to obtain any additional benefits to which she may be entitled, such as income support, housing benefit and council tax benefit, and any domicilary care services she may need. However, in order to benefit from the full range of services that are likely to be available in your area, Sarah or her neighbour may need to make contact with a local voluntary organisation, such as a community advice centre or Age Concern.

The impact of the community care reforms

At the time of the implementation of the NHS and Community Care Act in April 1993, Dr Brian Mawhinney, the then Minister of Health, stated 'We must not expect too much too soon. Benefits will flow from these reforms over a decade ... Success will depend not so much on this year's implementation agenda, but more on the continued vision of what can be achieved to allow people to live with independence and dignity.' While it is still too soon to evaluate the effectiveness of the community care changes, you are no doubt aware of the disquiet expressed by many health and social care providers, as well as service users and carers, about the shortcomings of the new arrangements for the delivery and funding of services. As Davis (1993) observes, attitudes to community care reflect the values that society holds for people who are disadvantaged by age, ill-health or disability and one of the main criticisms is that inadequate levels of public funding and provision are undermining the ideal of community care that meets the real needs and wishes of service users and those who care for them. One of the principal concerns, for instance, is the inadequacy of measures to support carers who will continue to provide the bulk of care in the community. Another major concern is the lack of support for people with mental health problems who have been moved from long-stay mental health units into the community, many of whom have become homeless and sleep rough each night.

In addition, the government's measures to limit public spending while, at the same time, encouraging the expansion of publicly-funded private services, contain many contradictions and make planning and budgeting increasingly difficult for local authorities and health authorities. Kingman (1994) points out, for example, that the private sector has been less than enthusiastic about expanding into the provision of domicilary services which are more difficult to supervise and manage than those provided in one building; they also require staff to work irregular hours, with peaks in the mornings and evenings when people need help getting up or going to bed. She also refers to the problems associated with the purchase of respite care from the private and voluntary sectors, citing a local organisation that admits it is nervous of committing more resources to this area because the social services department is unable to guarantee how much it would use such a facility.

From the perspective of both service providers and service users, there remains deep confusion about the extent to which community care is free. If a service is provided by a local authority or voluntary organisation, it is increasingly likely to be charged for. If it is provided by the NHS, it remains free. In many cases, however, it is often difficult to separate health and social care. A client who has suffered severe brain damage as a result of a car accident, for instance, may be assessed as needing respite care in a specialist centre where he can receive appropriate therapy. The question of who pays for it, or how the local authority and health authority share the cost, depends on the way in which health care and social care are defined. In practice, it appears that health care is increasingly being defined very narrowly, which means that growing numbers of people receiving community care are being means-tested for the services they receive. Such is the confusion that the Health Secretary announced in August 1994 that, by 1996, local comunity care charters would be introduced in England that would make clear whether and when elderly and disabled people would be required to pay for care services.

It is clear that the mixed economy of welfare will continue to operate in the provision of community care, even though the debate about the most effective ways of providing and funding services will long continue. If you are interested in reading more about this area, you are recommended to read 'Problems for the mixed economy of welfare' by Johnson (1990) which provides an excellent synopsis of the discussion in this session. *The Community Care Handbook: The new system explained* (Meredith, 1993) provides a comprehensive guide to the community care reforms and Davis (1993) assesses the likelihood of the reforms achieving the government's stated objectives.

In the next four sessions, we shall look in more detail at the role of the four main sectors in the mixed economy of welfare and consider the advantages and disadvantages of each of them.

Summary

1 The system of welfare provision in which services are provided by the statutory, private, voluntary and informal sectors is known as the mixed economy of welfare. The role of the statutory sector encompasses direct service provision and the funding, regulation and co-ordination of welfare services.

2 Community care is designed to help people who need care and support to live with dignity and as much independence as possible in the community. It consists of a wide range of domiciliary, day, residential, nursing and respite care services.

3 With the implementation of the NHS and Community Care Act 1990 in April 1993, local authorities are required to shift to an 'enabling role' and, wherever possible, to commission services from the private and voluntary sectors.

Before you move on to Session Four, check that you have achieved the objectives given at the beginning of this session and, if not, review the appropriate sections.

SESSION FOUR

The statutory sector

Introduction

In this session, we shall explore the ideologies of the Conservative and Labour parties in relation to the role of the statutory sector within the welfare state. In doing so, we shall address some of the key debates that take place within the discipline of social policy, including the relationship between government expenditure and the economy, the effects of taxation on the work ethic and the efficiency of the welfare state.

Ideologies are not discrete and do not come conveniently packaged. In reality, there exists a continuum of different perspectives ranging from the far right to the far left, with the Conservatives, the Liberal Democrats and Labour falling somewhere in the middle. However, we need only focus on the central areas of this continuum in order to understand the impact of ideology on policy-making and implementation in the field of social policy. In this session, therefore, we shall compare the approaches of the two main parties in the UK, the Conservative and Labour parties, although you may also wish to consider the policies of the Liberal Democrats and other political parties in response to the issues raised in this session.

Session objectives

When you have completed this session, you should be able to:

- identify some examples of social policy that reflect specific political ideologies

- outline Conservative Party ideology on the role of the statutory sector

- outline Labour Party ideology on the role of the statutory sector

- discuss the advantages and disadvantages of universal and selective welfare provision.

Ideology and social policy

In the political context, the term 'ideology' refers to the values, beliefs, ideas and theories that underpin the political views of each party and that are reflected in their policies. Despite the diversity of opinions held by Members of Parliament within each of the major parties in the UK, it is possible to isolate a range of views that can be said to dominate in terms of defining party policy. It is these that are referred to as the dominant ideologies.

You are no doubt aware of some of the major policy differences between the two main political parties. Central to Conservative economic policy, for example, is the importance of controlling inflation. In order to achieve this, they argue, there should be minimum government intervention in the economy and the supply and price of goods and services should be determined by market forces. Accordingly, the government has attempted to reduce public expenditure and has promoted competition and private ownership through such policies as the privatisation of nationalised industries, the reform of trade union law, tax incentives for businesses, encouragement of wider share ownership and compulsory competitive tendering of local authority services. In contrast, the economic strategy of the Labour Party is based on a policy of active involvement and investment by government, working in partnership with the private sector. This it believes, will result in significantly lower levels of unemployment that will in turn stimulate economic growth and increase government revenue because the number of people receiving benefits will fall and the number of taxpayers will increase.

These different views about economic policy are clearly reflected in the parties' views on social policy and on what they believe to be the most appropriate role for the state in the provision of welfare services. In the 1950s and 1960s, there was general consensus between the two major political parties about the role of the welfare state, which was seen initially as synonymous with the statutory sector, and the need to increase government spending. The three Conservative governments between 1951 and 1964, for example, presided over a rapid expansion in education and council house building. Since the election of the Conservative government in 1979, however, there have been shifts in the positions of both parties as the concept of the welfare state has come to be defined as the mixed economy of welfare. With the growth of mass unemployment and the concomitant growth of poverty, accompanied by periods of recession, the cost of the welfare state has grown substantially so that it now accounts for over a quarter of the gross domestic product, more than double the levels of the 1960s. The views of the two parties now diverge on the issue of whether the role of government should be to provide only minimum services for those with the greatest needs in society through a safety-net approach or whether it should reduce the demands on the welfare state by promoting a greater degree of social justice through an egalitarian or redistributive approach. Their differing views on the functions of the welfare state and how it interacts with economic policy directly influence the social policy responses that they advocate and their strategies for providing services.

Community care, for instance, is an area of social policy in which there is general agreement between the Labour and Conservative parties on many of the core principles involved. Both share the aim of preventing unnecessary institutionalisation and bringing more choice, more independence and better care to individuals and families in need. They also agree that community care services should be provided within a mixed economy of welfare and that there is a role for all four sector providers. Where they disagree, however, is on what they perceive the precise role of each sector to be within the mixed economy. As we have seen, the Conservative Party places particular emphasis on the role of the private, voluntary and informal sectors as the main service providers and is moving towards a minimal or residual role for the statutory sector. For the Labour Party, the state should retain a key role in the direct provision of services rather than merely being their purchaser, regulator or co-ordinator. Its policy on community care (1992) specifically states that:

> 'Labour will provide a level playing field between different providers so that the choice between public, private or voluntary care homes is not influenced by differential access to benefits. Labour is in favour of choice. We will oppose monopolies of provision, whether public or independent.'

The aim of the following activity is to encourage you to think about the two parties' policies in relation to two further areas of social policy and about how they reflect a broader political view or ideological position about the role of the state in the provision of welfare.

ACTIVITY 16   ALLOW 10 MINUTES

The Conservative and Labour parties have quite different views about the degree to which individuals should take responsibility for themselves and their families and on the role of the state in providing economic and social support. Try to identify some policies in relation to housing and health care that reflect these contrasting views.

Commentary

For Conservatives, the opportunity to own a home and pass it on to the next generation is one of the most important rights that an individual has in a free society and lies at the heart of their philosophy (Conservative Party, 1992). The expressed desire of the Conservative government to create a home-owning democracy is illustrated by its introduction of the 'right-to-buy' scheme for council tenants in 1980, which was subsequently extended by reductions in the qualifying period and the discounts available and by the introduction of the rent-to-mortgage scheme and the do-it-yourself shared ownership scheme. It actively encourages the expansion of the private rented sector and has transformed the role of the statutory sector in housing provision by restricting the amount of revenue from the sale of council housing available to local authorities, promoting the management of council housing by the private sector and the transfer of council properties to housing associations.

The Labour Party has accepted the right of council tenants to buy their homes and is now examining ways in which it could be extended to private tenants and more housing association tenants. However, it places far greater emphasis on the responsibility of the state to provide housing for those who cannot, or choose not to, buy their own home. For the Labour Party, housing is a national asset for which there must be a real measure of community responsibility and people should be able to choose the form of tenure that best suits their needs and income at each stage of their lives. Thus, the role of local authority housing is not merely to provide a safety-net for individuals who are unable to buy because of unemployment or low income or who cannot obtain housing in the private rented sector. Rather, it is an alternative form of housing tenure that enables people to have access to good quality, secure housing at an affordable price.

Both the Labour and Conservative parties express support for the NHS and the principle of health care that is free at the point of use. The introduction of tax relief for employers on employees' private health insurance by the Conservative government demonstrates its clear encouragement, however, for individuals to provide for themselves rather than relying on the NHS. Similarly, some of the provisions of the NHS and Community Care Act 1990, with its emphasis on the family's role in providing for their dependents and a shift from free service provision to the means-testing of some services, indicate the growing application of the safety-net principle. More broadly, the introduction of the internal market into the NHS with the separation of the purchasers and providers of health care and the growing role of the private sector in the provision of services reflect Conservative economic ideology about the best means of achieving an efficient and cost-effective service. As we have seen in Session Two, the Health of the Nation strategy focuses firmly on cultural and behavioural causes of ill-health with its emphasis on individuals' responsibility to lead more healthy lifestyles.

The Labour Party sees the Conservative focus on commercialisation and competition in health care as a means of preparing for the privatisation of the health service. For them, quality health care is about co-operation rather than competition and the NHS should therefore put patients before private profit and respond to the needs of the community in such a way that there should be no need for private health care provision. Labour views the internal market as resulting in an explosion of costs and bureaucracy rather than improved patient care and believes that the introduction of GP fundholding has created a two-tier system that enables some doctors to get preferential access to services for their patients and undermines the principle of equal access for equal need. Central to its strategy for health is its recognition of the impact of structural factors on avoidable illness and its commitment to wider social policies to achieve full employment, sufficient income, decent housing, a nutritious diet and protection from pollution as a means of improving health. Significantly, its policy document *Health 2000* is subtitled 'The health *and* wealth of the nation' (Labour Party, 1994).

Despite some criticism that the 'modernised' Labour Party of the mid-1990s is moving closer towards the principles of the Conservative Party, its policies are based on very different ideologies. As we progress through this session, we shall look in greater detail at the different social values, beliefs and theories that form the basis of the parties' dominant ideologies, and assess their importance in determining social policy. We shall begin by looking at the ideology of the Conservative Party.

The Conservative perspective

The Conservative party came to power in 1979 with a commitment to opportunity, choice, ownership and responsibility. It set out to achieve these goals through policies to promote competition and the free market and to cut public expenditure and reduce state intervention. This antagonism to the dominant role of the state is known as anti-collectivism because it reflects opposition to the notion that the state, as the representative of society, should take collective responsibility to provide for those in need unless they are genuinely unable to meet those needs for themselves. The Conservative critique of the welfare state and its commitment to limit the role of the state in the provision of welfare services is based on a number of grounds, but we shall focus on the four main interlinking arguments here:

- the welfare state undermines the economy

- it encourages dependency and discourages individual effort

- it is unresponsive to people's needs

- it is inefficient.

Undermining the economy

It is the argument that the welfare state undermines the economy that is crucial to our understanding of Conservative ideology. A central belief within this ideology is that high economic growth will generate sufficient wealth to enable the majority of the population to make their own provision for the welfare services that they want and need. Whilst recognising that social inequality is inevitable in a free market economy, this is considered to be both natural and, to some extent, desirable in that it functions as an incentive for people to work harder. In acknowledging that it is by no means a perfect system, Conservatives maintain that it is still the best system available. Their criticisms that the welfare state directly undermines the economy are based on the following arguments.

First, the burden of taxation required to finance the welfare state reduces the amount of money available to individuals, businesses, banks and building societies to invest in the economy. In other words, an ideology that supports large-scale state spending on social policy requires a policy of high taxation to finance it. If people are heavily taxed, their choices about how to spend their money are restricted; they may not, for example, be able to buy their own home, make provision for their retirement or pay for health care or education services of their choice. As a result, they place greater demands on the welfare state. The expansion of the private sector, needed for the achievement of higher economic growth, has also been undermined by the heavy demands of a taxation system that has placed it beyond the economic reach of most individuals.

Second, the incentives for tax-payers to work harder and earn more are reduced by attempts to promote social equality through a progressive tax system that is based on the principle of 'the more you earn, the more tax you pay'. So, taxing high earners heavily in order to finance a growing welfare state reduces their motivation to improve productivity that will contribute to greater national wealth.

Third, the demands on the welfare state have grown so much, partly because of the large increase in the elderly population, that its scope has become much greater than its inventors ever envisaged. In its present form, it is an economic burden that the state can no longer support. In 1992–93, for example, expenditure on social security benefits amounted to more than £74 billion, of which nearly half was accounted for by payments to elderly people. Social security benefits were the second most important source of income after wages and salaries (Central Statistical Office, 1994a).

Dependency

Conservatives also argue that the state has played such a prominent role in the provision of welfare services that the concept of self-reliance has been weakened. As a result, a dependency culture has developed in which people have neglected their own responsibilities to provide for themselves, their families and their communities. As Margaret Thatcher declared in 1984 in a speech to the Small Businesses Bureau (quoted in Andrews and Jacobs, 1990):

> 'I came to office with one deliberate intent: to change Britain from a dependent to a self-reliant society; from a give-it-to-me to a do-it-yourself nation; a get-up-and-go instead of a sit-back-and-wait-for-it Britain.'

Conservatives argue that a system of generous social security benefits and welfare provision discourages many low-income people from working because their needs are already being met through the state. They may, for example, have a council house, receive housing and council tax benefits, unemployment benefit or income support and free school meals for their children. Thus, the dependency culture encourages 'welfare scroungers' and undermines what are the natural and best sources of welfare: the family, voluntary action and the private market. As Ranade (1994) observes, Conservatives emphasise that 'Families owe responsibilities to each other, and for humanitarian and religious reasons the duty of charity to others. State welfare, it is claimed, undermines both kinds of obligation.' In the words of Michael Portillo (reported by Wintour, 1993) who is widely seen as the leading figure on the Conservative right:

> 'For many people, the role of government has sapped from them – one might almost say confiscated – their sense of responsibility towards other people. It's hard to be neighbourly if we are told the state should look after our neighbours ... While most people want to work, there are those who use the system to avoid it and for them the benefit culture becomes a way of life. That in turn demoralises those struggling to provide for themselves ... It's hard to be responsible within our families if we are told that the state should educate our children, teach them right and wrong and for that matter care for our elderly relatives. We end up by virtually renouncing any responsibility for the way our society develops, for its customs and morals.'

Furthermore, it is argued, many of those who want to work and improve themselves are often better off claiming welfare benefits. In effect, they are caught in a 'poverty trap' whereby any financial gains from working are undermined because they lose social security benefits on a pound for pound basis and they also become liable to pay tax.

This view of dependency has most recently manifested itself in the belief, now widely held, that Britain is seeing the emergence of a so-called 'underclass' which is characterised by its slothful behaviour and dependence on state benefits. Murray (1994) terms this the 'New Rabble'.

ACTIVITY 17   ALLOW **10** MINUTES

What policies introduced by the Conservative government since 1979 attempt to address its concerns about the effects of the welfare state on the economy and its role in creating a dependency culture? Try to identify at least five.

Commentary

Even though it introduced the biggest tax rise in the post-war period in the November 1993 budget, the Conservative Party has always claimed to be the party of low taxation. Its policy of lowering direct taxation and extending indirect taxation through VAT on goods and services is designed to give people more choice about how and where they spend their income. By extending tax relief to certain private sector services such as pensions and health insurance, it also encourages investment as a means of both stimulating economic growth and reducing dependency on welfare services. The lowering of the rates of taxation for high income-earners is similarly designed to stimulate economic growth by restoring financial incentives that will generate higher productivity, and hence higher profits, as well as releasing a greater proportion of people's income for savings and investment.

In addition to attempting to root out benefit fraud, the government also aims to ensure that people take more direct responsibility for their lives. The establishment of the Child Support Agency, for example, was specifically designed to shift the financial support of children in lone parent families from the state to their fathers, although its critics point out that it is the state, rather than the children, who benefit from higher maintenance payments. Incentives such as tax relief have promoted investment in private pensions that will reduce the number of elderly people requiring income support and other welfare benefits, while curbs in unemployment, invalidity and sickness benefits, the removal of earnings-related supplements to benefits, the axing of income support for 16–17-year-olds and the provision of retraining programmes are all designed to encourage people to return to work.

Unresponsive to needs

Conservatives also argue that the welfare state is unresponsive to the needs of those it serves and that many statutory welfare services tend to be overly bureaucratic and run more in the interests of those who provide the services rather than of those who use them. As a result, service users are often forced to tolerate standards that they would consider unacceptable in their private purchasing decisions. These problems could be overcome if services become more recipient- or consumer-led, as in the private market. Hence, the concept of the service user as a customer to whom service providers must respond has become a fundamental principle in the Conservative approach to the delivery of services. The Citizen's Charter, for example, was specifically developed to address the needs and extend the rights of those who use public services by requiring services to set clear standards and to tell the public how far they are being achieved.

In health care, for example, the length of waiting lists for hospital treatment has for long been a major source of dissatisfaction for patients. In 1991, the Department of Health published *The Patient's Charter: Raising the standard* which sought to put the Citizen's Charter into practice in the NHS in an attempt to make health services more efficient and responsive to patients' needs. The Charter outlined seven existing rights and three new rights, including a commitment to reduce waiting times to a maximum of two years. It also set national charter standards in nine key areas and emphasised the importance of local charter standards. Although the charter standards are couched in the language of 'rights', the Charter clearly states that they are not legal rights but important, specific standards that the government requires NHS hospital and community services to achieve.

Nevertheless, Conservatives argue that however much improvement is achieved in the quality and responsiveness of services such as the NHS, the monolithic nature of the public sector means that service users have little choice about the level or type of services that they wish to consume in order to meet their individual needs. Just as in the supermarket the consumer is able to choose from amongst a range of products, so too should the individual be able to choose from a range of welfare services. Thus, policies such as tax incentives for private health insurance and personal pensions and subsidies for grant-maintained schools are designed to promote competition between service providers that will result in greater individual choice, customer-led rather than provider-led services and quality in provision.

Inefficiency

The statutory sector is criticised by Conservatives as being inefficient, partly on the grounds of its unresponsive nature which results in many real needs not being met, but also because of its monopoly of many services which results in a lack of innovation and experimentation. This, it believes, inevitably leads to stagnation and a decline in the range and quality of services provided. The government's attempts to improve the efficiency of public services has led to dramatic changes in the way in which they are now planned and delivered. Fundamental to the reform of services ranging from the NHS to British Rail are the principles of competition and accountability. As John Major said in a speech to the European Policy Forum in July 1994: 'We are letting competition and choice into the public sector as a spur to efficiency ... Competition has a wonderful habit of concentrating the minds of those between whom a choice might be made.'

Accordingly, private companies are encouraged to bid for public sector contracts through compulsory competitive tendering for such services as community care services, local authority housing management and, increasingly, for central government services. Competition is also encouraged within the statutory sector, most notably in the NHS where the function of paying for care has been separated from that of providing care. District health authorities and family health services authorities have been merged to form purchasing commissions which are allocated funding on the basis of their resident populations. They can purchase services from their own local hospitals and community services, self-governing hospitals, private hospitals and community services or hospitals in any other health district. Fundholding GPs are similarly able to purchase a defined range of services from NHS or private provider units. The rationale for the internal market is that health care providers who offer efficient, cost-effective and high quality services will thrive, while those failing to do so will not survive.

The Conservative perspective on the welfare state thus centres on a belief that too much state intervention in welfare provision undermines what its supporters feel are central social values and institutions – economic growth, work incentives, the family, voluntarism and individual choice. Yet, despite these criticisms, Conservatives do see a role for the statutory sector in providing a safety-net welfare service that meets the needs of those who are poorest and a compulsory minimum education. Beyond this minimal role for the state, however, Conservatives look to the private, voluntary and informal sectors to provide innovative, high quality, cost-effective and responsive welfare services.

It is perhaps important to point out that the views that we have referred to as 'Conservative' are those that have been dominant within the Conservative Party since 1979 and that represent their view of what the role of the state should be. While the nature and extent of statutory provision within the welfare state has been under attack during this period from what is often referred to as the new right, the statutory sector remains largely intact, albeit with a somewhat different role. It could be argued, however, that this is mainly due to political expediency. The popularity that the NHS enjoys, for example, would lead to electoral suicide for the Conservative government if it openly challenged the basic principle that health care should be free to all at the point of use.

The Labour perspective

The Labour Party does not share the Conservative Party's faith in the free market as the best means of generating economic wealth and providing welfare services and, in particular, highlights the extent to which it leads to greater social and economic inequality. It is its emphasis on equality and social justice that is central to an understanding of the Labour Party's views on social policy. While the party has moved some distance away from its traditional focus on state ownership and control since the mid-1980s under the leadership of Kinnock, Smith and Blair, it firmly asserts the need for active government, working closely with business to invest in the future rather than leaving everything to the market.

Its social policies reflect its recognition that the welfare needs of today cannot be met by the welfare state of fifty years ago – or even of 1979 when the Conservatives took office. As a result, there has been a shift away from the traditional 'Levellers' approach of the old left, where the focus was on increasing benefits to alleviate poverty, to an approach that is based on investment in people to assist self-improvement and self-reliance and where citizenship is about matching rights and responsibilities.

For Labour, the key principles are social justice, opportunity, responsibility and trust and a belief in the ethical and moral superiority of collective welfare provision. Without government intervention, it believes, unemployment rises and social inequalities increase; not only does this contribute to lower economic growth and higher welfare expenditure, it also limits many people's freedom to participate fully in society and increases the potential for alienation and social conflict. Thus, social policy should not simply react to and compensate for economic policy, but should be creative and preventive in its function of overcoming poverty and promoting equal opportunities for all citizens. In practice, this means removing inequalities in areas such as health and education through active government intervention in social welfare.

For Labour, then, the state plays an important role in the promotion of social justice and equality and it seeks to achieve this through redistributive taxation and welfare policies designed to correct the failures of the free market. This approach, which has become known as the Labour Party's Strategy For Equality (Tawney, 1981), has four main aims:

- to ensure the supply of basic necessities to all
- to supplement income from work with services according to need
- to encourage economic growth through the improvement of people's health, education and general well-being
- to promote social justice and equality of opportunity.

The welfare state and the economy

Central to the achievement of these aims is a progressive and fair taxation system in which those with higher incomes pay a higher percentage of their earnings in tax than those on lower incomes. Labour favours taxes on income rather than on spending which, it argues, bear most heavily on the poorest sectors of the population while vastly increasing the disposable income of the rich. Thus, the extension of indirect taxation, such as the imposition of VAT on essential services such as domestic fuel, actually limits choice for many people, particularly elderly people and others on low income. Labour stresses the inherent contradiction in the Conservative contention that high income-earners need financial incentives to make them more productive, while unemployed people need financial disincentives to get them back to work and points out that successive tax changes under Conservative governments since 1979 have resulted in the majority of the population paying higher taxes, with the richest paying less. An analysis of the budgets since 1985 by the Institute of Fiscal Studies (cited by Elliott and Kelly, 1994), for example, divided Britain's 20 million households into ten groups and showed that the poorest four bands were all worse off on average from the cumulative tax changes, while the top six bands gained, particularly the top 1% of earners who saw their post-tax incomes boosted by 10%. At the other end of the scale, the poorest 10% of households saw a 3% reduction in their much smaller incomes. Furthermore, Labour asserts, the cost of tax evasion and perks for higher income-earners is far greater than that of benefit fraud and closing the loopholes in taxation policy will generate substantial additional revenue that can be invested in welfare services such as education, health care, housing and social services.

The Labour Party sees unemployment both as a major constraint on economic growth and an unneccessary drain on welfare resources and its social policies are therefore directly linked with its strategies to reduce unemployment. The phased release of local authority receipts from the sale of council housing, for instance, would enable more homes to be built and this would both contribute to the resolution of the housing crisis and revive the building industry. Thus, in contrast to the Conservative Party which has cut or restricted eligibility for benefits such as unemployment, sickness and invalidity benefits as part of its strategy to reduce unemployment, the Labour Party would set benefits at levels that would enable people to meet their basic requirements while, at the same time, investing in the creation of wider employment opportunities that reduce the need for people to claim those benefits. This, it is expected, will increase revenue from taxation and reduce demands on the state, thus freeing more welfare resources for others in need.

Labour supporters dismiss the charge that welfare expenditure and a redistributive taxation policy undermines the economy by depriving it of the investment required to create wealth for the nation. They maintain that progressive taxation is a form of investment in all people and that it is only by maximising and building on the talents and abilities of everyone within society and ensuring social stability that the country's economic potential can be increased. Thus, they believe that better working and living conditions improve the quality and productivity of labour and go hand in hand with economic prosperity. As part of its commitment to equality and social justice, for example, the Labour Party sees the Social Chapter as representing both a set of social standards to which every civilised industrial nation should aspire and a step towards economic renewal and is thus committed to anti-discriminatory practice and equal opportunities policies.

The following activity asks you to think about Labour's view that large-scale government intervention in social policy is a necessary investment in society.

Note down at least two ways in which you think that the welfare state works to maximise talent by 'investing in people'.

Commentary

Labour believes that active government is often essential to enable people to take greater control over their own lives. It is committed to working towards full employment, a national minimum wage and fair employment practices that would enable people to live with dignity and independence in a society in which their contribution is valued and respected. It believes that Britain's future lies in high-skill, high-quality jobs, not in cheap labour and poor working conditions that force many people into a reliance on the welfare state. It therefore supports the Social Chapter with its commitment to equal rights for part-time, full-time, temporary and permanent workers, including equal pay and access to paternity leave. In addition, its focus on the structural factors that contribute to inequalities in health will, it is expected, contribute to a healthier, productive nation that will make fewer demands on the NHS and community care services. Its proposals for the state provision of nursery education for all children under the age of five are designed both to improve educational standards and opportunities for the workers of the future and to enable more women to rejoin the workforce. As Harriet Harman (1993), Labour's shadow Treasury Secretary argues:

'Government action to ensure the availability of childcare and job opportunities would transfer single parents, for example, from the public spending side of the balance sheet and help them to emerge on the revenue side, as taxpayers. This is the classic case where government action will enable people to provide for themselves rather than having to depend on other taxpayers . . . We do not think that the best government is the biggest government. But there is public support for active government partly achieved through public spending. This approach would bring about economic regeneration and assist every individual to reach their full potential. It would turn public spending from a palliative for economic failure into a springboard for economic success.'

The extent to which the modern Labour Party sees the need for economic efficiency to go hand-in-hand with social justice is illustrated by its positive response to the report of the Commission on Social Justice, an independent body set up by the late Labour leader, John Smith, under the auspices of the Institute for Public Policy Research (1994). Although the report, *Social Justice: Strategies for national renewal*, was not intended to be a manifesto for the Party, it was described by Smith's successor, Tony Blair, as undoubtedly the most significant and comprehensive analysis of the welfare state since Beveridge and a major challenge to the governing philosophy and ethos of the previous fifteen years of Conservative rule. The report proposed a radical programme of social and economic reform in key areas such as employment, pensions, child benefit, education and housing and in smoothing the path from welfare to work through strategies to promote full employment, the introduction of a minimum wage, the development of a modern social insurance system and a reform of the main means-tested benefits such as income support. As Blair argued in a speech at the launch of the report:

'A more just society should allow us to invest in the areas we wish to spend on and cut the areas of spending that are merely the consequence of social decay ... A successful economic policy combined with effective modern welfare would mean a reduction in the benefit bill ... Social justice is about building a nation to be proud of. It is not devoted to levelling down. Or taking from the successful and giving to the unsuccessful. It is about levelling up.'

Efficiency and quality

Conservative criticism of the statutory sector as being unresponsive, overly bureaucratic and inefficient is largely shared by the Labour Party, which agrees on the importance of achieving higher standards in public services. It accepts that services could and should be more client-oriented, but does not consider this problem to be insurmountable. Indeed, it believes that it is not necessarily related to state provision, but is more a feature of large organisations, be they public or private. It argues that the problem could be resolved by making welfare organisations smaller, located within the communities which they serve, and more accountable to the local people who use them by allowing the general public more control in the way the services are provided. Thus, while the Labour Party supports the local management of schools, a policy introduced by the Conservatives, it opposes the centralised control of school budgets through the Funding Agency for Schools which it considers to be an unaccountable, unfair and wasteful Quango (quasi-autonomous non-governmental organisation). It also resists health authorities and hospital trusts being placed in the hands of unelected government appointees, many of them Conservative party supporters who have no experience of the NHS.

The Labour Party's broad approach to improving the quality of services is summarised in its strategy for health (1994):

'Labour intends restoring the principle of a National Health Service which puts the patient before private profit and which responds to the needs of the community. We want to see a health service which is effective, efficient and fair. Market-driven competition leads to an uneven distribution of facilities and services across the country, while commercialisation of health provision wastes resources on unnecessary bureaucracy. Quality health care is about co-operation not competition ... The Tory obsession with privatising and commercialising health care has resulted in an explosion of running costs, at the expense of improved patient care. They have dramatically increased waste, reduced openness and accountability and damaged the morale of those working in the service ... Our objective is that everyone is able to receive free treatment, equal access to the service and fast, effective redress where necessary. Labour's NHS will be accountable to the whole of the local community, not to accountants and government appointees.'

Thus, Labour does not envisage a major role for the private sector because, in its view, welfare services should exist to meet need, not to make a profit, and should be provided according to need rather than individuals' ability to pay. It sees voluntary organisations as playing an essential role in welfare provision, but as a complement to public services rather than as a substitute for them.

Selectivity and universality

One of the most obvious differences between the two main political parties is to be found in their policies on how welfare resources should be distributed. The traditional Conservative view of a safety-net welfare service has, as its basic principle, the targeting of benefits and services at individuals who are most in need. This selective provision relies on means tests to check whether claimants meet a specified level of poverty or need that would render them eligible to receive a particular service. Income support and family credit are examples of benefits provided on a selective basis.

In contrast, the Labour Party maintains that some forms of welfare service should be provided on a universal basis: that is, that they should be available to all. Child benefit is an example of a universal welfare benefit that was introduced by a Labour government specifically to tackle the problem of child poverty. Thus, every family with children is eligible for the benefit without having to prove that its income falls below a certain level. Although the Conservative government has not abolished this benefit, it has eroded its value by failing to update it in line with inflation. The principle of universality relies on a progressive taxation system to recoup the benefits paid to the more affluent in society; with wealthy recipients of universal benefits paying more through taxation than low-income families to finance those benefits.

The aim of the following activity is to encourage you to think about the problems associated with these two diverse approaches to welfare eligibility.

ACTIVITY 19 — ALLOW 15 MINUTES

There are two welfare benefits that are aimed at overcoming child poverty: child benefit which is based on the principle of universality, and family credit which is based on the principle of selectivity. Using these two benefits as examples, what do you think are the advantages and disadvantages of the universal and selective approaches to welfare benefits?

You may find it useful to study the procedures for applying for child benefit and family credit before you complete this activity. Child benefit and family credit packs are available in all post offices. You might like to complete the claim forms to get an impression of the processes involved in assessing eligibility.

Commentary

There are three main arguments against selectivity based on means tests, such as that applying to family credit, and in favour of universal benefits such as child benefit. Firstly, the means test may deter people from applying for benefits because of the complexity and intrusive nature of the questions asked to establish eligibility. Many potential recipients are too proud and independent to claim the benefits to which they are entitled because the tests require them to declare themselves as being poor. As a result, selective benefits often fail to meet their objectives of helping those most in need because the take-up rates are low. The provision of free school meals on a selective basis to children whose families are demonstrably poor is an example of how means-testing can stigmatise individuals and may result in poor take-up by those in need. Secondly, rather than targeting resources on those most in need, means tests are in practice often used to limit the demand for services or benefits. In other words, they constitute a crude rationing device. Thirdly, an emphasis on means-tested benefits and services creates a social climate in which the recipients are negatively viewed as a burden on society.

For these three reasons, means-tested benefits and services tend to be under-used. Oorschot (1991) examined social security benefits across Europe and found that the take-up of benefits that are not means-tested is very high in the UK, with the proportion of people claiming benefits such as child benefit being close to 100%. The study showed that, in contrast, the take-up of means-tested benefits was much lower, with only about 23% of those eligible claiming housing benefit and 46% claiming family income supplement, the predecessor to family credit.

A fourth objection to selective benefits based on means tests is, however, that they are extremely expensive to administer. In some cases, the administration costs involved in assessing who is eligible, and who is not, may be as high as 30% of the total expenditure allocated to the benefit. It is for these reasons that the Labour Party favours the universality principle, as with child benefit, which they see as being more cost-effective to administer and which has a high take-up rate because it is not used to limit demand and has no stigma attached to it.

The main argument against the universality principle and in favour of selectivity is that universal benefits are taken up alike by those in need and those not in need. Wealthy families, for example, are entitled to the same amount of child benefit as the poorest of families. The payment of universal benefits to all is therefore an unneccessary drain on finite resources. This forces taxpayers to pay more for wasteful services that should, instead, be targeted on those with the greatest needs. Equally importantly, the availability of universal benefits encourages a benefits culture that robs people of their independence and discourages them from making provision for their own needs and taking responsibility for their lives. Although it is accepted that the take-up of selective benefits is much lower than that of universal benefits, it is argued that the solution is to improve access to information to ensure that those who are genuinely in need will know they are eligible and will apply for the appropriate benefits.

As we progress through Sessions Five to Seven, the extent to which the two dominant ideologies are reflected in the social policies of each party will become clearer. This should enable you to assess the implications of each party's policies, not only for the direct recipients of social welfare but also for the wider society.

Summary

1   Dominant ideologies within each political party in the UK have important implications for what they consider to be an appropriate role for the state in the provision of welfare services.

2   Conservative ideology demands that the state should have only a limited role in welfare provision, that individuals are the best judge of their own needs and interests and that the market is the most appropriate provider of welfare services. Conservatives criticise the post-war welfare state on the grounds that it undermines the economy, creates a dependency culture, is unresponsive to individual needs and is inefficient.

3   In contrast, the Labour Party stresses the importance of collective or shared responsibility and the harmful effects of social and economic inequalities. It maintains that the market is not the best provider of welfare services and that it is the role of the state to promote social justice through a progressive taxation system which redistributes resources and finances welfare services.

4   The Conservative Party supports the principle of selectivity in welfare provision in order to target benefits and services on those in greatest need. The Labour Party places greater emphasis on the provision of benefits and services on a universal basis.

Before you move on to Session Five, check that you have achieved the objectives given at the beginning of this session and, if not, review the appropriate sections.

The private sector

Introduction

In the last session we explored the contrasting views on statutory provision of welfare services held by the Labour and Conservative parties. We saw that the Conservative Party emphasises the primary role of the family and of private and voluntary provision and argues that the state should concentrate its welfare resources on those whose needs are greatest and cannot be met by these other sectors. In contrast, the Labour Party emphasises the role of the statutory sector as the principal provider of social welfare within the mixed economy of welfare and supports the notion that the state can and should play an important role in the promotion of equality through the distribution of welfare services.

When it came to power in 1979, the Conservative Party embarked on the longest period of single-party rule in the post-war period. As a consequence, the main thrust of social policy during the 1980s and early 1990s has been a growing shift of responsibility for the provision of social welfare on to the private, voluntary and informal sectors. We shall consider the implications of this for the voluntary and informal sectors in Sessions Six and Seven. In this session, however, we shall focus on the advantages and disadvantages of increasing reliance on the private provision of public welfare by examining the influence of private sector provision and values in the areas of housing and health care.

Session objectives

When you have completed this session, you should be able to:

- assess the impact of the shift towards private sector provision on the role of the state

- identify the advantages and disadvantages of the emphasis on home-ownership in contemporary housing policy

- discuss the implications of the growth in private health care and the introduction of the internal market to the NHS for consumer choice, the quality of services and equality of access.

The shift to private sector principles and provision

The Conservative belief in free market principles and its firm encouragement of private enterprise and market values has underpinned the government's attempt to 'roll back the state'. We have seen how Conservatives view the private sector as being superior to the statutory sector for the following reasons.

1   The private sector gives welfare recipients – or consumers – a greater degree of choice about the type of welfare services they use.

2   It is also more responsive to their demands because, in the market-place, the customer is sovereign. The market will always provide for consumers who wish to buy a certain product or service – and have the money to back that desire – because it exists to make profit and can only do so by responding to their wishes. This profit motive is arguably lacking in the statutory sector where consumers have little power to determine the nature and availability of services.

3   As a consequence, the private sector is more efficient at meeting needs because competition to meet consumer demands directly shapes the services that are provided and they are not mediated by professionals who may have their own, rather different, views about what a person's needs are.

The impact of this Conservative ideology on British society has been wide-ranging, not least on the welfare state where the most tangible effects have been:

- increased incentives for people to use the private sector and disincentives for them to rely on state-funded services

- a growth in direct service provision by private suppliers

- the introduction of private sector values, models of management and patterns of financing in the statutory sector.

We have already explored the way in which Conservative government policy explicitly encourages people to take more individual responsibility for providing for their own welfare needs. Here, we shall consider the impact of the growth of private sector provision and approaches in two of the areas where it has become most evident:

- housing

- healthcare.

The private sector in housing

The area of social policy most affected by government encouragement of the private sector over the last twenty years or so has been that of housing policy. As we saw in Session One, housing can be provided in a range of different ways and, in the UK, is provided through four main 'tenures':

- owner-occupation or home ownership

- local authority accommodation

- private renting

- voluntary housing associations.

The largest area of growth has been that of the private home ownership sector which has been actively encouraged by both the Labour and Conservative parties through policies specifically designed to help owner-occupiers, such as mortgage interest tax relief and renovation grants, and fiscal policies designed to maintain low interest rates. Other policies assisting low-income home-owners include such Labour government initiatives as the option mortgage scheme, which was designed to give non-taxpayers the same tax relief as taxpayers. It is, however, the Conservative Party that has largely been responsible for a massive shift to private ownership and a decline in renting. The introduction of the right-to-buy programme under the Housing Act 1980 and its Scottish equivalent gave all local authority tenants the right to buy their own homes, with generous discounts, if they had been tenants for more than three years. The maximum available discount was raised from 50% to 60% in 1984 and then, in 1987, to 70% for flats. By the end of 1992, more than two million public sector tenants had made applications to buy their homes, with nearly seven in ten actually making a purchase. Annual sales peaked at 200,000 in 1982, with a smaller peak in 1989, although only 65,000 were sold in 1992 (Central Statistical Office, 1994a).

In 1983, the government introduced the rent-to-mortgage scheme, enabling council tenants who had not been able to buy their homes to take a part-share in them, gradually stepping up to full ownership. It also established the do-it-yourself shared ownership programme, enabling first-time buyers to choose a home and buy a share of it, usually 50%, and pay rent on the rest to a housing association until they wish to increase their stake in the property.

The success of government schemes designed to expand the role of the private sector through increasing owner-occupation can be seen clearly by the fact that, by 1992, more than twice as many homes were owner-occupied than in 1961, as shown in *Figure 8* which illustrates the increasing significance of home ownership compared to the number of homes rented from local authorities, housing associations, privately or with a job or business during the period 1961–1992.

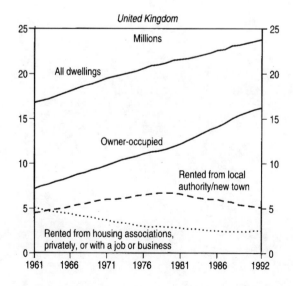

Figure 8: Stock of dwellings, by tenure, 1961–1992
(Source: Central Statistical Office, 1994a)

The right to home ownership and to pass it on through inheritance is a fundamental principle in Conservative ideology. Its policy to shift ownership of council housing into the hands of individuals is also supported on the grounds that it has freed tenants from the control of overly-bureaucratic local authority housing departments. Tenants are now able to do what they wish with their own homes. They can sell them and buy in a different area, decorate them according to their own taste or install new front doors, bathrooms or kitchens. As the new owners of their own homes, Conservatives believe, former council tenants become more self-reliant and take more responsibility for meeting their own housing needs. Apart from the immediate advantages to those who have bought their council homes, however, what have been the wider consequences of the right-to-buy scheme?

ACTIVITY 20   ALLOW 10 MINUTES

In what ways do you think that the right-to-buy scheme has affected those households in housing need who have *not* been able to take advantage of the scheme?

Commentary

The vast majority of the 1.5 million council homes sold in the 1980s and early 1990s under the right-to-buy scheme were those of the highest quality – typically semi-detached houses with gardens on popular estates. It proved extremely difficult for local authorities to sell the poorer quality housing which remained, particularly the large number of high-rise flats. Some tenants could not afford to buy or were not eligible for mortgages because of their low income, unemployment or age, although the rent-to-mortgages scheme is designed to enable low-income council tenants in employment to buy their homes. Others chose not to buy because of fears about the future resale value. As a consequence of the nature of the properties sold and the government freeze on new council house-building, the right-to-buy scheme has resulted in a residue of poor quality, unpopular council properties often situated in unattractive, stigmatised parts of our towns and cities.

Unfortunately, the Conservative government's expectations that the shortfall in council house-building resulting from the freeze would be made up by new private sector housing have not been fulfilled. Although private enterprise now dominates housebuilding, accounting for over 80% of new homes, it built only 125,000 houses and flats in 1992 compared with 138,000 in 1976 (Central Statistical Office, 1994a). Historically, the private sector has never been a supplier of decent, low-cost housing for those on low or irregular incomes because, quite simply, there is little profit in doing so. The deepening recession of the early 1990s and consequent increases in unemployment have further reduced the numbers of houses built in the private sector, resulting in an ever-increasing gap between the number of houses available and the number of households requiring them.

Even though building by voluntary housing associations is making up some of the shortfall, the decline in local authority housing stock has meant that many who cannot afford to buy or rent privately or do not have access to housing association schemes now face considerable difficulties in finding suitable housing and many young couples are unable to set up home together at all. It is perhaps significant that the tensions created by housing shortages have been identified by local people as a key factor in the rise of groups such as the British National Party, which achieved short-lived success in local elections in the Isle of Dogs in 1993. The shortage of affordable housing has also been a major contributory factor in the increase in homelessness. In 1986, 118,000 households were accepted as homeless; by 1992, this had risen to 167,000 with a further 90,000 households applying to a local authority who were found not to be homeless and 6,000 who were judged to be intentionally homeless. *Figure 9* illustrates the dramatic increase in the number of homeless households in England who were housed by local authorities in temporary accommodation during the period 1982–92.

England				Thousands
	Bed and breakfast	*Hostels*	*Short life Leasing*	*Total*
1982	1.6	3.5	4.2	9.3
1983	2.7	3.4	3.7	9.8
1984	3.7	4.0	4.6	12.3
1985	5.4	4.7	5.8	15.9
1986	9.0	4.6	7.2	20.8
1987	10.4	5.2	9.2	24.8
1988	11.0	6.2	12.9	30.1
1989	11.5	8.0	18.4	37.9
1990	11.1	9.0	25.1	45.3
1991	12.2	10.0	37.8	59.9
1992	7.7	10.7	44.5	62.9

Figure 9: Households in temporary accommodation, 1982–92
(Source: Central Statistical Office, 1994a)

During the same period, the number of people housed by local authorities from the ordinary waiting list declined, mainly because of the increase in the number of homeless people in defined categories of 'priority need' whom they are required to help. Contrary to the government's expectation that the informal sector will play an increasing role in welfare provision, the most common reason why people become homeless and require accommodation from local authorities is that parents, relatives or friends are no longer willing or able to accommodate them (Central Statistical Office, 1994a).

Recession and other recent economic developments have also highlighted some of the disadvantages of relying on the private housing market to meet housing needs. High unemployment and fluctuations in interest rates have affected many home-owners, including many ex-council tenants, and this has led to unprecedented numbers of repossessions. The Central Statistical Office (1994a) reports an increase from 4,900 repossessions by mortgage lenders in 1981 to 75,500 in 1991, although this fell to 68,500 in 1992. As a consequence, many people who have had their homes repossessed now find themselves homeless but ineligible for rehousing in even the poorest council accommodation because local authorities do not have a statutory responsibility to rehouse former owner-occupiers.

Ironically, the government has failed in its attempt to reduce public spending on housing policy because the steady rise in owner-occupation has increased the number of people eligible for mortgage interest tax relief. Between 1961–62 and 1990–91, the cost in real terms to the government increased tenfold to £8.3 billion, as shown in *Figure 10*, although there was a substantial drop in 1992–93 because of a fall in interest rates and a reduction in tax relief.

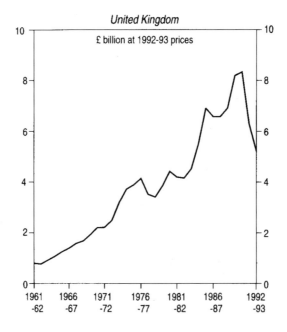

Figure 10: Total real cost of mortgage interest tax relief
(Source: Central Statistical Office, 1994a)

How successful do you think the housing policy of the 1980s and 1990s has been with its strong emphasis on home-ownership? To what extent has this improved choice? How efficient has it been in responding to housing need and demand?

Commentary

Using the government's own criteria, we can see that the private housing market is efficient in providing choice for those who can afford it, but is unable to cater for demands placed on it when the economy is in recession. Providing housing for those on low incomes is unprofitable and it is for this reason that the private market does not respond to their demands, with their needs largely remaining unmet. As a result, there is very little choice for some groups in our society. It is not surprising, therefore, that housing tenure is so closely related to the household's socio-economic position, with rates of home-ownership being lowest in low-income groups, as *Figure 11* illustrates.

Great Britain			Percentages
	Owned with mortgage	Owned outright	Rented
Professional	72	15	13
Employers and managers	77	13	11
Intermediate non-manual	69	11	20
Junior non-manual	58	15	27
Skilled manual	61	14	25
Semi-skilled manual	42	13	46
Unskilled manual	29	17	54
Economically inactive	10	43	47

Figure 11: Tenure by socio-economic group, 1992
(Source: Central Statistical Office, 1994a)

The government has not simply confined its transformation of housing tenure to home-ownership, however, but has also demonstrated its determination to encourage a strong private rented sector. This is subsidised through housing benefit for people living in rented accommodation who have insufficient income to be able to afford the full rent and there are plans to introduce a rent-a-room scheme under which home-owners will be able to let rooms to lodgers without having to pay tax on the rent they receive. The encouragement of the private sector far goes beyond this, however. As part of its strategy to revolutionise the management of council homes, the government has introduced compulsory competitive tendering to bring in private sector providers operating on contract to local authorities. As a result, many people are offered accommodation that has been arranged by the local authority and is leased from private landlords rather than permanent accommodation in council homes. Tenants often have little security of tenure since, if a private landlord goes into receivership, there is no guarantee that the tenancy will be maintained. Although standards and inspection procedures are often rigorous, there are fears that the spectre of Rachmanism – landlords who charge extortionate rents for slum properties – will re-emerge. Indeed, a growing problem for local authorities is that they bear the cost of housing benefit but cannot control the rents charged by private landlords, which are set at market levels.

The private sector in health care

As in housing, the private sector has become increasingly important in the provision of health care services. The private provision of health care is not new. Many people have long chosen to use complementary therapies such as homeopathy, medical herbalism and acupuncture for which they have to pay. Private nursing homes existed well before the NHS was established and expenditure on private health care has been rising since the 1970s. The number of authorised beds in NHS hospitals for private in-patient care has declined, but there has been an explosion in the provision of registered private nursing homes, hospitals and clincs, as shown in *Figure 12*.

Mohan (1991) argues that the rhetoric of privatisation has not been matched by radical policy changes in health care because the government White Paper, *Working for Patients* (Department of Health, 1989) that led to the major reforms of the NHS in 1990 departed relatively little from the original objectives of the

England			Thousands and percentages	
	1971	1981	1986	1991-92
NHS hospital authorised beds for private in-patient care (thousands)	4.5	2.7	3.0	..
Registered private nursing homes, hospitals and clinics Total available beds (thousands)	25.3	31.9	62.1	147.2
Percentage of available beds in premises with an operating theatre	..	..	14.5	6.5

Figure 12: Private health services: number of beds
(Source: Central Statistical Office, 1994a)

NHS, at least in terms of its comprehensiveness, public funding and the absence of charges at the point of use. The reforms that were introduced under the NHS and Community Care Act 1990 transformed the organisation of health service funding and delivery through the separation of the purchasing and providing functions which freed purchasing commissions to buy services from private as well as NHS provider units. Nevertheless, as Mohan suggests, in contrast to other areas of social policy such as housing:

> 'There has been no national renunciation of a commitment to the availability of comprehensive health care. Instead, there has been a questioning of the legitimate scope of state activities.'

It is important to bear in mind the political and electoral considerations that the government has had to bear in mind, given widespread public support for the National Health Service. Opinion polls, for example, consistently show that any attack on the fundamental principles on which the NHS was founded would result in a massive loss of political support. You may find it interesting to read 'Disquiet and welfare: clinging to Nanny' by Taylor-Gooby (1989) which provides a useful discussion of public attitudes to welfare. However, although the material impact of the White Paper, in terms of privatisation, may not have had a major impact on the availability of services, its ideological influence in setting the context for future developments cannot be underestimated.

Two aspects of privatisation are important in relation to recent developments in health policy:

- the aim of mobilising private provision in order to supplement state provision, particularly in the areas of residential care and nursing homes and private medical insurance

- the introduction of private sector management styles and approaches within the NHS.

Private residential care and nursing homes

The changing age structure of the population has clear implications for the demand on welfare services and is one of the key reasons why the government fears that the state will be increasingly unable to afford the costs of providing welfare benefits and services for everyone. This supports their view that their needs are best met through other sectors and that, as far as possible, people should make their own provision for their retirement rather than relying on the state. In 1961, just under 12% of the population were aged 65 or over. By 1991, nearly 16% were in this age group and the proportion is projected to rise to just over 22% in the year 2031. By 2001, nearly 10% of households will comprise a man living alone, while women over pensionable age are expected to form the largest group of one-person households, at around 11% of all households (Central Statistical Office, 1994a). Laing and Buisson (1993), the independent health care consultants, estimate that 1.5% of the gross domestic product is currently spent on long-term nursing care for elderly people, three-quarters of which is raised from taxation. By 2050, the figure is predicted to rise to 3.5%.

Part of the government's strategy to cope with the demands of an ageing population is to shift the responsibility for welfare from the state to the private sector and, with a potentially enormous market for private residential and nursing care, provision has increased considerably since the 1970s. This growth was aided by a change in the benefit rules in 1983 when the government allowed elderly people living in private residential care to claim their fees from the then Department of Health & Social Security. This contributed to a rapid increase in both the number of private residential homes and the number of people living in them. There were 1,871 private residential care homes in 1975, but this number had grown to 9,235 in 1992. During the same period, the number of private nursing homes rose from around 1,000 to more than 4,000 (Laing & Buisson, 1993). Under the community care reforms in 1993, responsibility was shifted from the Department of Health to local authorities for assessing the type of care required and for paying some or all of the fees for private residential care. With the requirement under the NHS and Community Care Act 1990 for local authorities to commission residential care services from the private sector in preference to the statutory sector, the opportunities for private sector providers are greatly increased. As Davis (1993) comments:

> 'The boom in residential and nursing homes during the 1980s was a response to the financial gains to be made through investment in these businesses, which coincided with a rapidly increasing market because of demographic change. But the majority of private homes would not have opened to admit the large numbers of people needing care unless public funds had been available.'

One justification for the policy to use public funds to pay for private care is a consumerist one – that of providing increased choice for elderly people. Andrews (1984) suggests, however, that it is private homes that are able to exercise increasing choice in the selection of their 'customers', rather than the other way round. Whilst conducting a research study for Avon County Council Social Services Department on the provision of places for elderly people suffering from dementias, for instance, Ackers (1986) was informed by community psychiatric nurses of the policy of some residential homes to 'remove' clients who became incontinent or developed behavioural problems. The pattern of growth has also varied from region to region. The Audit Commission (1986) highlighted the tendency towards 'territorial injustice' (or geographical unevenness) that has resulted from the increasing reliance on the private sector for the provision of residential care. It found, for example, that there were nearly ten times as many places per 1000 people aged 75 and over in private and voluntary residential homes for elderly people in Devon and East Sussex than there were in Cleveland. While this can, in part, be explained by the fact that there is a higher demand in certain areas because many people choose to move when they retire, the fact remains that private provision is uneven and does not necessarily reflect the need for services.

We have seen how private sector growth in residential care and nursing homes has effectively been subsidised by the Department of Health and, since the community care changes in April 1993, by social services departments. This has important implications for the role of the state in the regulation and control of the private sector. Under the Registered Homes Act 1984, all residential homes for four or more people have to be registered. Health authorities are responsible for the registration and inspection of nursing homes, while local authorities register private and voluntary homes and inspect all residential care homes, including their own.

ACTIVITY 22   ALLOW **10** MINUTES

Imagine that you are planning to set up a private residential care home for elderly people. What aspects of your plans do you think would require approval before you could be registered by your local authority or health authority?

Commentary

The Residential Care Homes Regulations 1984 stipulate that local authorities must be sure that:

- the applicant for registration or any other person concerned with running the home is a 'fit person' to be involved with a residential home

- the premises are 'suitable' for the purpose of the home

- the way it is intended to run the home will provide the services or facilities reasonably required.

The law does not define a 'fit person' or 'suitable premises', so each local authority interprets the rules in its own way. The Regulations state that the person registered must run the home so as 'to make proper provision for the welfare, care and, where appropriate, treatment and supervision of all residents'. Meredith (1983) summarises the key requirements in terms of the facilities and services to be provided as follows:

- employment by day and, where necessary, by night of enough suitably qualified and competent staff to be adequate for the well-being of residents

- 'reasonable' day and night-time accommodation and space for residents

- adequate and suitable furniture, bedding, curtains and floor covering and, where necessary, equipment and screens in rooms used by residents

- adaptations and facilities necessary for physically disabled residents

- adequate light, heating and ventilation in all parts of the home used by residents

- maintenance of all parts of the home occupied or used by residents in good structural repair, clean and reasonably decorated

- regular laundering of linen and clothing

- arrangements, where necessary, for residents to receive medical and dental services

- suitable arrangements for recording, safe keeping, handling and disposal of drugs

- suitable arrangements for the training, occupation and recreation of residents.

Other factors that would need to be taken into account include the degree of disability of the proposed residents, which may involve decisions about the siting of the home and its proximity to main roads, residential areas and transport links. There may also be controls on the numbers of residents that you are permitted to accept. All these factors would affect the potential profitability of your proposed home.

The setting of standards and inspection is obviously crucial to protect the residents of all homes, whether private, voluntary or statutory. In fact, local authorities did not have to inspect their own homes until the NHS and Community Care Act 1990 was implemented, when they were required to set up inspection units. However, the regulation needed to ensure the safety and security of residents arguably undermines the independence of the private sector. As Mohan (1991) suggests:

> 'Although privatisation has meant that the state in one sense has been rolled back, then, the demands of regulation may require that it is rolled forward in another direction in order to protect the vulnerable.'

There was a strong reaction from health care professionals and the public against a letter from the Department of Health to proprietors of private nursing homes in September 1983 about a proposed radical review of regulation to assess the costs for businesses and identify ways of reducing the 'burden'. The proposal was quietly shelved. Concern is growing, however, about the number and nature of complaints against staff in private homes. Disciplinary hearings against nurses in private homes, for example, accounted for 26% of all cases heard by the United Kingdom Central Council for Nursing, Midwifery and Health Visiting in the first half of 1993 (Eaton, 1993) and the UKCC is concerned that although many homes are well-run, staff recruitment procedures are sometimes poor, there may be very little study leave or professional updating available and inspection units are often over-stretched.

Private medical insurance

In an attempt to encourage the use of private alternatives to the NHS, in 1985 the government offered tax incentives on private medical insurance to individuals and to employers who provide it for their employees. As a result, it is becoming increasingly common for employees' salaries to be topped up with membership of private medical insurance schemes such as those run by the British United Provident Association (BUPA), the Private Patients' Plan (PPP) or the Western Provident Association (WPA). The number of people with private medical insurance policies has grown steadily, increasing by about 50% between 1985 and 1990, although it fell by 1.7% in 1991, as shown in *Figure 13*.

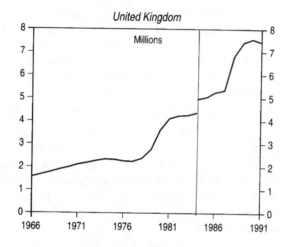

Figure 13: Private medical insurance: persons insured
(Source: Central Statistical Office, 1994a)

The government argues that private medical insurance offers individuals the opportunity to choose the providers of their health care and to change them should they be dissatisfied. This places providers in competition with one another which, it is expected, increases their efficiency and responsiveness. It may sound like an attractive argument for turning to private medical insurance, but how accurate is it? What are the problems of relying on the private sector to provide health care?

ACTIVITY 23   ALLOW **10** MINUTES

Do you or any other members of your family have private health care insurance? Why do you think people pay for insurance rather than using the NHS?

Commentary

The key reason why people choose to pay for private health care insurance appears to be that it offers reassurance and peace of mind, rather than because of concerns about the quality of services offered by the NHS. Promotional materials from the insurance companies invariably focus on the advantages they offer in terms of protecting against long NHS waiting lists and their high standards in medical facilities, comfort and service. The Norwich Union Healthcare policy, for example, is typical in its focus on prompt treatment:

> 'We all rely on the NHS, but although it's acknowledged as one of the best providers of hospital care in the world, especially for accidents and emergencies, there are long waiting lists for many types of treatment and operation. It simply cannot provide immediate care for everybody for all conditions. If you are suffering from a "non-urgent" complaint and need an operation, you could well face a long delay – possibly of over a year. Private Medical Insurance is a way of protecting you against waiting for an operation ... if you need in-patient or day-patient hospital treatment we will pay for you to have it in one of the "Select Hospitals".'

Many policies also provide cash benefits for people receiving hospital treatment to compensate for loss of income when they are unable to work. The recent growth in personal health insurance schemes, such as critical illness and income protection schemes which provide lump-sum payments and regular income during periods of serious illness, also reflects a trend away from reliance on state sickness and invalidity benefits which are set at a low level and for which more stringent criteria are being applied.

The argument that private health care is more efficient than the NHS does not seem to be borne out by the experiences of those countries in which the private sector is the dominant provider of health care. The administrative and financial costs involved in, for example, selling private medical insurance packages, examining doctors' bills and having to account for every penny spent are enormously expensive. In fact, the former Health Minister, Dr Brian Mawhinney (reported by White, 1993), justified the large increase in administrative staff since the introduction of the NHS reforms by reporting that administration costs accounted for 13% of USA health care costs, compared with only 2% in the NHS. It is significant that although health care in the States costs around double the proportion of the gross domestic product than in Britain, the USA has higher infant mortality and lower life expectancy than most developed countries, partly because health promotion and primary care have little place in the world of insurance.

For patients, the obvious disadvantage of private health care is its cost, which they have to bear on top of their contributions to the NHS through tax and national insurance. As a result, the majority of the population do not have access to it. Although the quality of private care is invariably high, some people express concern about the nature of the doctor–patient relationship in a profit-making situation. They fear that because few patients are knowledgeable about medical matters, they are in a vulnerable position in relation to the doctor who could recommend expensive and unnecessary treatment in order to increase their profits, as sometimes appears to happen in countries such as the USA where treatment and care are largely privately financed.

One of the major weaknesses of private medical insurance from the consumer's point of view, however, is that it is based on similar principles to all other insurance schemes, such as car and house insurance. Thus, the higher the risk of illness, the higher the insurance premium that the individual has to pay.Ultimately, there are some people whom private health insurance companies will not insure at all because they consider them to be a 'bad risk'. In practice, most companies only insure individuals who are at relatively low risk of illness and, even then, typically provide cover only for acute illnesses that can be treated by a short stay in hospital.

ACTIVITY 24 · ALLOW 10 MINUTES

What groups of people do you think might find it difficult to obtain private healthcare insurance? If private insurers will not provide for them, who will?

Commentary

Private healthcare insurance schemes typically include a range of limitations. In general, they will not accept new members over a certain age and members cannot claim for any current illness or previous medical conditions that originated in a specified period before joining and have not been cured. Most schemes do not cover certain health conditions, such as pregnancy, childbirth, infertility treatment, abortion and sterilisation, treatment for mental, addictive or allergic disorders, renal dialysis, HIV, AIDS and other sexually transmitted diseases and cosmetic surgery. In addition, the costs of seeing a GP privately, convalescent care, home help and nursing homes are often excluded from cover, as are the fees for private consultations with specialists that do not result in hospital treatment. There may also be a maximum limit on the sum that can be claimed to cover medical costs so patients requiring long-term treatment or care may be forced in the end to turn to the NHS. In practice, therefore, many people who might wish to take advantage of private health care have no alternative but to use the NHS.

For the NHS, a high proportion of the cost of direct health care is devoted to providing for the very groups whom private healthcare insurance excludes. Conservatives argue that the expansion of the private sector enables NHS resources to be directed at those most in need. However, there are some contradictions in this view because the private sector relies heavily on NHS resources and facilities in order to provide its services, including doctors and nurses who have been trained at state expense, authorised beds in NHS hospitals for private in-patient care and expensive equipment. These are all resources that could be used for NHS patients. In addition, the government subsidises private medical insurance through tax relief to employers. In practice, the expansion of the private sector is effectively leading to a two-tier health system, with one service for those who can pay and one for those who cannot. There are widespread fears that, as has been the case in the provision of housing, this will inevitably lead to a poorer quality NHS and that its users will ultimately face the problems of stigma that are associated with an inferior service directed at people who are poor.

The view of private sector provision as being *the* answer to the UK's health care problems is therefore open to question. As Davis (1993) points out, if public funding is restricted, the 'industry' could collapse, with catastrophic consequences for the NHS which still has an obligation to provide services. It is important to recognise, too, that the nature of health care is such that it must always be imperfect. There will always be a greater demand for health services than supply, for two main reasons. As the Department of Health indicates in *The Health of the Nation* (1992), life expectancy at birth has increased considerably and now stands at 73 years for males and 79 years for females. At the same time, the government's overall goal is 'to secure continuing improvement in the general health of the population ... adding years to life and ... life to years'. Clearly, further improvements in life expectancy and the quality of life will bring about increased pressure on health service resources.

The provision of health care is, then, by its very nature associated with the rationing of scarce resources and with decisions about which patients will be given priority. Under a system of private provision, rationing is achieved through the provision of services according to the ability to pay, which accounts for the 40 million Americans who have no health insurance. In the UK, rationing has effectively been carried out by the medical profession who decide whose needs are the greatest; this accounts for the NHS waiting lists. Since the 1990 NHS reforms, however, rationing is increasingly being determined by the allocation of resources, as demonstrated by freezes on routine surgery by health care provider units which 'fulfil their contracts' before the end of the financial year.

The influence of private sector management styles and methods

In addition to the expansion of private health care provision, it is important to recognise the influence of private sector approaches and models of management on the NHS. The stress on public expenditure restraint has led to demands for greater efficiency across all welfare sectors and many of the recent changes in the health service have been influenced by experience drawn from the private sector. As we have seen in Session Four, the major reforms heralded by the NHS and Community Care Act 1990 introduced an internal market into the NHS through the separation of the purchasers and providers of health care and opened up new opportunities for the private sector to provide services. This competitive approach was designed to improve the efficiency, cost-effectiveness and quality of health care. The influences of private sector principles were felt earlier, however, in 1984 with the introduction of NHS general management in line with the recommendations of the NHS Management Inquiry (Department of Health & Social Security, 1983). Its chairman, Roy Griffiths, appointed because of his experience as chairman of Sainsbury's and later knighted for his work, was highly critical of the previous style of NHS management and his views were crystallised in a famous sentence: 'If Florence Nightingale were carrying her lamp through the corridors of the NHS today she would, almost certainly, be searching for the people in charge.' The reforms proposed in the Griffiths Report were introduced in 1984 but, since 1990, there has been a further explosion in the number of management posts within the NHS, many of which have been filled by people from the commercial and industrial sectors.

The government White Paper, *Working for Patients* (Department of Health, 1989a), which led to the NHS reforms, specifically aimed to create a new NHS management culture, build a climate more favourable to private provision and open up new areas for private sector involvement both within and outside the NHS. It emphasised the importance of localism and local management in the provision of services in order to raise the performance of all hospitals and GPs to a high standard of efficiency and cost-effectiveness and many of the appointees to the executive boards of NHS trusts are specifically selected for their business expertise. Health service managers are able to draw on community resources, including charitable and commercial facilities and sponsorship schemes, and have greater freedom from national pay scales and from supervision by regional health authorities. NHS hospital trusts are able to borrow money on the capital markets and are allowed to generate surpluses or profits.

Despite the economic motivation for the government's strategy to roll back the state and expose more areas to competitive private enterprise approaches, however, its attempts to improve health service management have not yet been been effective in controlling public expenditure on health care. Indeed, the costs have continued to increase each year, as shown in *Figure 14*.

At the same time, there is little evidence to show that the expansion of private provision has reduced the demands on the public sector as private customers come off NHS waiting lists.

England			£ million at 1992-93 prices	
	1981-82	1986-87	1991-92	1992-93
Health authorities – current	14,388	15,561	18,821	19,878
Health authorities – capital	1,228	1,497	1,695	1,908
Family health services	4,616	5,222	6,223	6,640
Other health services	..	..	683	703
Departmental administration	..	..	270	316
Total cost of NHS services	20,861	23,050	27,694	29,445

Figure 14: National Health Service expenditure, by sector
(Source: Central Statistical Office, 1994a)

ACTIVITY 25

To what extent do you think that the expansion of the private sector will relieve pressure on the NHS by reducing waiting lists? Note down your ideas.

Commentary

Most private medical insurance schemes focus on the provision of in-patient hospital treatment and do not cover the full range of services offered by the NHS. Typically, the first step for a person covered by a private healthcare insurance policy involves going to see their GP, who is trained and employed by the NHS. The GP will decide whether they require referral to a specialist (again, trained and employed by the NHS) and will arrange an NHS appointment in the normal way. If the specialist then recommends in-patient or day-case treatment, they will find out how long the waiting list is. In most cases, only if the patient's condition is eligible for cover and the wait for the recommended treatment is more than a specified period, often six weeks, will the insurance company step in and either pay for private treatment to beat the queue or provide financial compensation for the wait. With some policies, if the waiting list is shorter, the member can claim a cash benefit on top of their treatment by the NHS.

It is not immediately apparent how much this scheme does to relieve the pressure on NHS resources, except by taking private patients off NHS waiting lists for non-emergency surgery. It merely prevents private patients from having to wait for long periods and gives them some cash compensation, which has little effect on NHS lists. So, although there may be some benefit to the NHS by private patients coming off long waiting lists, the relationship is not as clear as that envisaged by the government.

In terms of political goals, the growing role of the private sector in health care fits neatly into the concept of a society which envisages a residual role for statutory welfare services – a society in which the successful are rewarded through such benefits as occupational pensions and healthcare insurance schemes and the 'undeserving' are penalised for their failure through an enforced reliance on public sector provision. Mohan (1991) refers to the ideological effect of creeping privatisation '... in stressing the limits to state action and the necessity and desirability of individual and community effort. In this regard privatisation's most important role may be that of preparing the ground for far-reaching change.'

The effects of the NHS reforms are indeed far-reaching and will continue to have a direct impact on both the availability of services and their cost. Despite some clear improvements that have emerged, particularly in terms of the quality of the care that is provided, the Conservative government has a long way to go in convincing health care professionals and the public that the NHS is safe in their hands. In the forefront of opposition to many of the changes are the doctors, most of whom seem to concur with the views of Dr Sandy Macara, chairman of the British Medical Association, who called for an urgent reform of the NHS reforms in an impassioned speech to the BMA's 1994 annual meeting:

'Doubt not that there is despair in the air today. There is despair about the mood of alienation and demoralisation in the NHS ... Co-operation has been supplanted by commercial competition. There is an uncontrolled, ill-managed internal market pitting purchaser against provider, fund-holding GP against non-fund-holding GP, GP against consultant, junior against senior, hospital against hospital and all to serve a perverse philosophy of winners and losers. Business plans override clinical priority. Money does not follow the patient: the patient has no choice but to follow the money. Treatment, except in emergencies and one begins to see it even in emergencies, has become a national and local lottery. Slow tracking, not fast tracking, is the reality for far too many patients ... I'm not suggesting we turn back the clock but we believe we can reform the reforms in the interests of our patients. We want to restore services which are patient-sensitive rather than driven by an ideological imperative.'

The ideological battle about the role of the private sector and its influence on statutory provision will long continue to rage. In the next session, we turn to the voluntary sector which is similarly undergoing a major transformation in the welfare state of the 1990s.

Summary

1 The shift in favour of the private provision of services has resulted in a changing role for the state from being the main direct service provider to having a greater purchasing, regulation and co-ordination function.

2 In a welfare system dominated by private provision, those who are eligible and can afford it benefit from increased choice, but the private market is unresponsive to the needs of those who cannot pay and who therefore have little choice in their access to services. This accords with the Conservative concept of society in which inequality is both the norm and, to some degree, socially desirable and where the role of the statutory sector is to provide a safety-net service for the poorest and those in greatest need.

3 State provision that is limited to a residual welfare system does not necessarily lead to greater efficiency, cost-effectiveness, choice and responsiveness to needs.

Before you move on to Session Six, check that you have achieved the objectives given at the beginning of this session and, if not, review the appropriate sections.

SESSION SIX

The voluntary sector

Introduction

In this session, we shall examine the changing role of voluntary organisations in the mixed economy of welfare and the implications of the shift in the respective roles of the state and the voluntary sector. We shall consider some ideological and practical concerns about voluntarism and explore how the growth in service provision by voluntary organisations through the contracting of services is leading to some fundamental changes in their place in society.

Session objectives

When you have completed this session, you should be able to:

- describe the range and scope of voluntary sector involvement in the provision of welfare

- review some of the ideas and ideologies underpinning the expansion of the voluntary sector, in particular the notion of altruism or giving freely to others

- assess the role of voluntarism and its place within social policy

- suggest areas where voluntary sector involvement may be most appropriate.

The role of the voluntary sector

The term 'voluntary sector' is generally used to refer to charities, self-advocacy groups and other not for profit organisations that have been set up and largely run by volunteers under a management committee, although all but the smallest agencies generally employ some paid staff. The voluntary sector has always played an important role in the provision of welfare services, as recognised by Sir Roy Griffiths in his influential report on community care (1988) in which he identified the following key roles performed by voluntary organisations:

- self-help

- provision of information

- befriending

- advocacy

- public education

- campaigning

- innovation and monitoring.

Voluntary agencies vary considerably in both their level of specialisation and also in the kinds of activities they undertake, with some focusing on the delivery of services, others adopting a largely campaigning and educational role and some forming self-help and self-advocacy networks to support people with similar interests or needs.

Resource 7, Caring for Thousands (Women's Royal Voluntary Service, 1992), outlines the scope of activities in which just one long-established voluntary organisation is involved. In addition to its well-known role in providing meals-on-wheels services and running hospital shops, canteens and ward services, its activities range from supporting the emergency services to working with offenders and their families.

Voluntary organisations range from large national or international organisations with professional staff such as Save the Children and the Royal National Institute for the Blind to small, local groups that operate on a largely informal basis, such as those providing visiting and befriending services or running local youth groups. Not only is there great variety in the size and management structures of these organisations and their level of dependence on volunteers, there is also considerable diversity in their sources of funding, which has important implications for social policy.

Some voluntary organisations receive relatively little subsidy from the government, apart from tax relief on investments and covenants and other financial advantages such as council tax relief. Their funding may come from a variety of sources, including membership fees and subscriptions, donations from the public and from industry, and their business activities, such as charity shops and mail order sales of Christmas cards and other goods. Others are heavily funded by the government, either at local level by local authorities, including social services departments and health authorities, or directly by central government. As we have seen in Session Three, there has been a considerable shift from grant aid to the commissioning of services from voluntary organisations, particularly in health, social services and education, with many voluntary bodies becoming increasingly dependent on public sector contracts for which they must bid against private companies and consultants.

Despite the many differences between organisations within the voluntary sector, the common feature is that they rely heavily on voluntary effort, largely through the use of volunteer workers, particularly for fund-raising. *Figure 15* shows the membership and the number of branches of selected voluntary organisations in 1971 and 1991, which illustrates the scale of volunteer activity in the UK, much of it in the field of social welfare.

Great Britain				Thousands and numbers
	Membership (thousands)		Branches/ centres (numbers)	
	1971	1991	1971	1991
Age Concern England	..	180	..	1,100
British Red Cross Society	172	82	917	1,200
Confederation of Indian Organisations	.	.	52	82
Disablement Income Group	..	5	..	..
Lions Club of the British Isles and Ireland	8	21	302	897
National Association of League of Hospital Friends	250	240	835	1,220
National Association of Round Tables of Great Britain and Ireland	29	23	1,072	1,220
National Federation of Community Organisations	.	.	564	921
National Federation of Gateway Clubs	8	77	200	723
National Federation of Self-Help Organisations	.	.	400	2,500
National Society for the Prevention of Cruelty to Children	20	21	217	220
PHAB (Physically Handicapped and Able Bodied)	2	50	50	500
Retirement Pensions Association	600	33	1,500	600
Rotary International in Great Britain and Ireland	50	65	1,125	1,760
Royal British Legion	750	655	4,135	3,268
Royal Society for Mentally Handicapped Children and Adults	40	55	400	550
Royal Society for the Prevention of Cruelty to Animals's	..	21	207	207
St John's Ambulance Brigade	..	55	..	3,209
Toc H	15	5	1,046	412

Figure 15: Selected voluntary organisations: membership and branches, 1971 and 1991 (Source: Central Statistical Office, 1993a)

Voluntary sector involvement in welfare provision is valued not only because the use of volunteers reduces the costs of services, but also because voluntary organisations are often highly innovative and pioneering in their approaches to meeting the needs of service users. They invariably offer more flexible and specialist provision for client groups than statutory agencies and can provide for greater participation by the people they represent in their policy making and in the planning and delivery of services. While there is wide political agreement on the importance of voluntarism and the notion of self-help, the issue that has attracted much debate within social policy during the early 1990s is the role of the voluntary sector in relation to the statutory sector. What do you think are the advantages and disadvantages of increasing reliance on the voluntary sector in the provision of welfare?

ACTIVITY 26 — ALLOW 5 MINUTES

Note down at least two reasons why you feel that Conservatives favour the expansion of the voluntary sector and the Labour Party is reluctant to see it replace existing provision.

Commentary

An expanded role for the voluntary sector is a key element of Conservative ideology, with its support of the concepts of responsibility and citizenship and its rejection of the 'something for nothing society'. The government recognises the experience and expertise that many voluntary organisations have developed in working with particular client groups and their ability to respond in innovative ways to the needs they identify. It also attaches considerable importance to voluntary sector provision as a means of reducing public expenditure although, despite generally lower overheads, it is not necessarily more efficient or cheaper than statutory provision. Thus, as we have seen, it specifically requires local authorities to commission community care services from voluntary agencies as well as private agencies and sees them as playing a central role in the mixed economy of welfare.

The Labour Party, with its philosophy of collectivism, agrees that voluntary organisations have an essential role to play in welfare and, in some settings may be appropriate agencies to manage relevant public services. It fears, however, that the distinctive contribution that they can best make in developing innovative, pioneering schemes will be put at risk if they are forced into being mainstream providers substituting for direct provision by the statutory sector. It also points to the danger that a greater reliance on voluntary organisations might absolve government of its responsibility not only to address people's needs, but also to remedy the structural problems that give rise to them in the first place. In its policy on community care (1992), for instance, it states:

> 'We do not believe that voluntary activity is either a threat, or a cheap alternative, to the provision of statutory services and any attempt to make it so should be resisted in the interest of both agencies. This is particularly important in relation to dependent older people, the mentally ill and those with learning difficulties. Most voluntary agencies spend much of their energy lobbying for more, not less, public sector provision and have no wish to be used as the excuse for a reduction in the public effort. Labour offers voluntary agencies a new partnership within an effective community care programme to meet the needs of the people whom we both serve.'

Labour's fear that a major expansion of voluntary provision could undermine statutory services and, in some cases, eventually replace them derives not only from its ideology on the role of the state, but also from its concern that it may be difficult to ensure uniform and high quality services through the wider use of volunteers who may not be adequately trained. Some Labour supporters also argue that expansion of the voluntary sector would directly threaten the jobs of professionals working within the welfare state. Can you think of any areas of nursing and social work which could be undertaken by volunteers? What do you think might be the implications for the employment of health and social care practitioners and ultimately for patient and client care?

Altruism

One of the most powerful arguments for the promotion of voluntary action and charitable giving is that it encourages people to face up to their responsibilities as citizens instead of simply looking to the state to meet their own needs and those of others. This argument is firmly supported by the Conservative Party and is grounded in the major religions which stress the importance of philanthropy and individuals helping each other in building caring and responsible communities. This Good Samaritan ideal has been widely debated by social philosophers who have used the concept of altruism to explain society's attitude to voluntarism.

Ware and Goodin (1991) define altruism very loosely as 'behaviour that benefits another (unrelated) actor and which imposes some cost on the originator'. In its purest form, voluntarism constitutes the giving of someone's time or resources without the expectation that they will be reimbursed in some way. Perhaps the best known research on altruism in social policy is that undertaken by Titmuss (1973) on blood donation. He explored public attitudes towards the giving of blood, which he interpreted as an act of altruism or a gift to an 'unknown stranger', by conducting a comparative study of the system of voluntary non-remunerated (unpaid) blood donation in the UK and the system involving the payment of donors and various contractual arrangements which operated in the USA at the time of his research. He concluded that the UK system fostered a system of welfare founded on altruism, whilst that in the USA encouraged the development of a society based on payment and self-interest. What are your own feelings about giving blood?

ACTIVITY 27

Have you or members of your family ever given blood? Why do you think that people give blood voluntarily and what might be some of the disadvantages of paying blood donors?

Commentary

Titmuss found that practically all of the voluntary blood donors he surveyed in the UK used a moral vocabulary to explain their reasons for giving blood, acknowledging a freely accepted responsibility to look beyond their own immediate needs and gratifications. He found that 'To the philosopher's question "what kind of actions ought we to perform?" they replied, in effect, "those which will cause more good to exist in the universe than there would otherwise be if we did not so act."' Thus, people who give blood on a voluntary basis do so because they feel that it is morally right and because they want to be able to help to save the lives of other people. Titmuss found, however, that none of the donors were purely altruistic because they also saw blood donation as a form of insurance. Thus, they expected that if they, in turn, needed blood in the future, adequate supplies would be available because others would also donate. Nevertheless, because there could be no certainty that they would need it or even that it would actually be available, their actions constituted a free gift that was given for the greater good without any conditions. The strength and extent of public willingness to give is demonstrated by the effectiveness of the blood transfusion service in the UK which has never had to offer financial incentives in order to maintain an adequate supply of blood.

In contrast, Titmuss concluded that the commercialisation of blood and donor–recipient relationships in the USA had clear negative effects in ethical terms because it repressed the expression of altruism, eroded the sense of community, increased the danger of unethical behaviour and exploited the mainly poor, unskilled and unemployed people who sold their blood in order to generate income, often at the expense of their own health. As he observed, 'Redistribution in terms of blood and blood products from the poor to the rich appears to be one of the dominant effects of the American blood banking systems.' He also found that, in non-ethical terms, commercialised blood donation was economically and administratively inefficient, more costly, resulted in gluts and shortages and compromised the safety of the patient because of the increased risk of transmission of infection from the donor. Since Titmuss published his study, the American system has been radically reformed and now relies on voluntary, unpaid donors.

Ware and Goodin (1991) believe that 'pure altruism' – or the gift to 'the unknown stranger' – is unlikely to survive in Western societies, dominated as they are by capitalism and individualism. They suggest, however, that what is more likely to remain is 'reciprocal altruism', which is really a form of exchange, entered into on the basis that a person who assists another within a wider reciprocating group may expect to receive similar assistance in the future, if required. Abrams (1977) had earlier come to a similar conclusion that altruism in contemporary Western society is typically self-centred and suggested that 'although we cannot hope to build on spontaneity (spontaneous "giving") as a basis of community care, we may well be able to build on reciprocity.'

ACTIVITY 28 — ALLOW 5 MINUTES

Why do you think so many people donate money or give their time to voluntary organisations? Note down your ideas.

Commentary

People who share their financial resources, their time and their skills with others obviously have a range of motivations. Many people join voluntary organisations because of their desire for justice, social change and equality of opportunity and their vision, commitment and belief in the worth and dignity of others. For many who donate to charity, participate in fund-raising or undertake voluntary action, the motivation may be 'pure' in the sense that they have no expectation of any personal return in the future, particularly where the organisation is concerned with overseas emergency or development aid. It could perhaps be argued, however, that their actions constitute a form of reciprocal altruism in the sense that they derive emotional benefit from the satisfaction and pleasure of sharing with others. For others, voluntary involvement also offers an opportunity for personal development and enables them to develop skills and experience that may be of benefit in future careers. Much reciprocal altruism operates on an informal basis, such as local baby-sitting circles in which parents do not pay for the service they receive, but provide the same service for others. Other examples include car-sharing for journeys to work or helping someone with their shopping or gardening when they are ill in the knowledge that they would do the same in return.

Ware and Goodin (1991) also consider the implications of what they call the 'institutionalisation of altruism' – the development of large-scale charities, often nationally or internationally organised and managed. They argue that, as charities expand, the gap between the donors and the recipients of charitable support ever increases; they become distanced to such an extent that individuals are unable to see the connection between their contributions and the results and, consequently, many become disenchanted and less likely to give in the future. Fund-raising campaigns which focus on the sponsorship of individual children, with the sponsor receiving photographs and regular feedback on 'their' child's progress, are an obvious example of attempts to lessen this distance.

Voluntarism

Voluntarism is heralded by the Conservative Party as a morally superior form of behaviour which preserves the principle of free choice because people are not compelled to give as they are via taxation, but can choose when and how to give – either financially through donations to charities of their choice or through voluntary effort. In 1981, for instance, Margaret Thatcher (cited in Waine, 1992) demonstrated her support for the increased role of the voluntary sector in a speech in which she declared:

> 'I believe that the volunteer movement is at the heart of all our social welfare provision. That the statutory services are the supportive ones underpinning, where necessary, filling the gaps and helping the helpers.'

Ware (1991) points out, however, that there is some contradiction in the arguments of the political right in relation to voluntarism, given its over-riding support for the market economy and the expansion of market-led and privatised forms of welfare. He argues that, while it may be agreed that voluntarism can be a useful means of controlling public expenditure and might be expanded on that basis, the overwhelming message coming from successive Conservative governments of the 1980s and 1990s is the notion that we only get what we pay for and that the competitive nature of the private market is the best means of achieving efficiency, quality and cost-effectiveness in welfare services. He therefore questions whether the notion of meeting needs through altruism – through voluntary action – is compatible with a predominant market basis for social organisation, concluding that the introduction of market forces into the welfare state actually tends to erode altruism.

Ware also argues that the expectation that increasing affluence will result in greater philanthropy, or voluntary giving, will not necessarily be met. In the USA, for example, total contributions to charity between the 1930s and 1950s increased from only 1.5% to 2% and after that did not increase at all (Ware, 1991). Attempts by the Conservative government to boost charitable giving through the Payroll Giving Scheme and tax relief on gifts and bequests have similarly met with limited success. Indeed, according to the Charity Households Survey, the typical donation per household in the UK was as low as £1.28 per month in 1989–90, a figure that was lower than each of the previous two years (Waine, 1992). There are increasing signs of compassion fatigue in the public's response to the proliferation of charity fund-raising and emergency appeals, particularly because of the level of economic hardship and uncertainty during the recession of the early 1990s.

At the same time, many companies are adopting a more hard-nosed approach to charitable giving and are increasingly linking donations to their business interests. A survey undertaken by Corporate Citizen magazine (cited by Brindle, 1994a) showed that corporate donations to charity declined in 1992–93 for the first time in more than ten years. The 100 leading corporate donors together gave £105.6 million, £2.4 million less than in the previous twelve months, although the figures relate only to cash gifts and exclude other support for the community. As the magazine's editor commented, 'Gone are the days of philanthropy. Sponsorship is favoured by companies who want their pound of flesh.'

It is clear that the concept of voluntarism that is seen as being necessary to underpin any extension of the role of the voluntary sector rests on idealistic assumptions about human behaviour and attitudes which may, in reality, not exist. Apart from questions about the level of altruism and support for voluntarism that exists in contemporary society, however, there are other practical concerns about the viability of increasing reliance on the voluntary sector, including:

- the funding of voluntary provision and the extent to which it should be provided by central or local government or supported by charitable fund-raising

- the need to regulate voluntary sector provision to ensure that services are of high quality and conform to government standards

- potential unevenness in voluntary sector provision, including the need to ensure that different parts of the country and groups of people with similar needs are equally well-served.

Financing voluntary sector provision

It is recognised that the steady replacement of many areas of statutory provision with voluntary sector provision will require higher levels of public funding and that, without it, the voluntary sector will be unable to become the major provider of welfare that is envisaged. *Figure 16* illustrates the extent to which many charities are dependent on voluntary income and the pattern of giving.

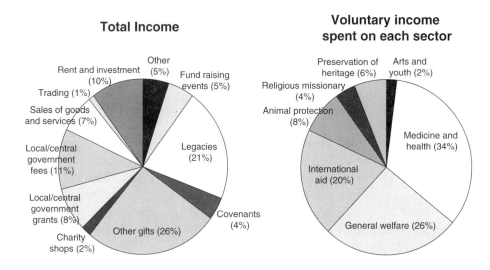

Figure 16: Total income and voluntary income of selected charities, 1990
(Source: Central Statistical Office, 1993a)

The transfer of money from the statutory sector to the voluntary sector may not, in itself, result in a reduction in public expenditure. Indeed, it is possible that losses in the economies of scale that can be achieved by large-scale providers such as local authorities may actually result in increased overall costs. It may no longer be possible, for example, to maintain a centralised transport network or to provide central kitchens for the production of food for school meals or meals-on-wheels. Each individual scheme may therefore have to make individual arrangements, such as contracting private transport, resulting in increased costs overall.

Despite government commitment to expand the voluntary sector, the contracting of services may actually serve to discriminate against some voluntary organisations. They are increasingly having to compete for public support and as more and more employ professional fund-raisers to generate income, the pressure on small groups means that some may not be able to survive without state funding, even though they may be highly effective. Many are finding that the continuation of general grant funding is being linked to their agreement to contract for services. This poses a dilemma for those that do not wish to change or expand their role or be part of the 'contract culture', but are dependent on local authority funding for some or all of their work. As Meredith (1993) observes, 'Contracting is a complicated process, involving legal responsibilities on both sides. Some small organisations will have neither the expertise nor the resources to deal with this. They are worried that they might be overlooked completely if authorities tend to turn towards larger organisations to contract services, perhaps reducing or cutting altogether their grants to other organisations. This has already happened in some areas.' Brindle (1994b), for example, cites the concerns expressed by the director of Home-Start UK, a charity offering support and practical help to families to prevent crisis and breakdown: 'There is a curious anomaly that at the very time when some local authorities are increasing their funding to established schemes, others are having to cut their grant to voluntary organisations, including Home-Start ... The problem is that we are a small voluntary organisation, with overheads already pared to the bone, and if they cut our funding – they kill us.'

Regulating voluntary sector provision

Injections of state funding into the voluntary sector may be necessary to ensure its viability, but may also impose serious constraints on its ability to respond to needs with organisations increasingly having to tailor their projects to meet the objectives and contract specifications of bodies awarding grants and contracts. On the one hand, state regulation is essential to ensure acceptable standards of care but, on the other, there are widespread fears of it being yet another erosion of independence and autonomy that may choke innovation and reduce many organisations to a sterile and dependent role. As Meredith (1993) points out:

> 'If voluntary organisations are increasingly expected to contribute to the "mixed economy of care" by becoming service providers, there are some worries that their ability to act as independent observers of public policies and innovators of new types of care may be reduced. If they have a large contract with the local authority to provide one service, will they be able to comment on some other aspect of the local authority's policy without endangering the contract on which they depend? If they must follow the local authority's priorities in order to obtain a contract, they may have to neglect innovatory or less high priority schemes which may have been the main reason why they were set up in the first place.'

Government pressure can certainly be brought to bear on voluntary organisations to curb their campaigning activities. In 1992, for example, Oxfam was warned by the Charity Commissioners that some of its activities were 'too political' and that, if these activities continued, it risked losing its charitable status. It is possible, however, that the voluntary sector may become subject to more widespread controls on their activities, as in the Netherlands, where the government has increasingly made use of financial pressures to impose rationalisation and quality control on the voluntary sector (Johnson, 1990).

A vision of how this approach might be dramatically extended in the UK came with the publication of a controversial report *Voluntary Action* (Knight, 1993) for the Home Office, which was the most comprehensive review of voluntary organisations since Beveridge's special report on the voluntary sector in 1948. The report proposed that voluntary organisations should lose their charitable status, their tax concessions should be withdrawn and the Charity Commissioners should be abolished. Voluntary organisations would then be divided into two separate categories. The first category would contain non-profit service providers, mainly the large voluntary organisations already bidding for contracts in the new purchaser–provider markets emerging in health, social services and education. These would be fully funded by the state. The second category would contain organisations that would return to their traditional role of campaigning, education and piloting new ways of delivering services. These would receive no state funding, but would depend on private donations from charitable trusts, foundations, industry and individuals. The report sent shock waves through the voluntary sector, not least because of its damning indictment of many of the larger organisations which, it says, have lost their vibrancy, energy and strength as they have become more dependent on state funds and insufficiently independent to warrant the description 'voluntary'. Although the report's proposals were not implemented, they serve as a reminder of how its central place in the mixed economy of welfare is necessarily changing the nature of the voluntary sector.

The precarious position of many charities was further reinforced by the Duke of Edinburgh when, in a speech in June 1994, he initiated a debate about the scope of charities and the benefits they receive. He suggested that the current definition of charitable status is too broad, attracting all and sundry 'like a magnet' with its promises of tax breaks, and proposed that charitable status should be restricted to strictly humanitarian causes.

The funding and regulation of voluntary organisations by the state also raises some important questions about the issue of accountability. It can be argued, for example, that local authorities that provide services are accountable to their local communities through the electoral process. This means that if they spend too much or too little, or spend inappropriately, they can be voted out of power in the next election. Voluntary organisations receiving state funding are not subject to the same kind of controls, although they are accountable to their members and to the public who finance their work. Leat (1987) identifies three potential problems in relation to the accountability of voluntary organisations funded by public money. These include accountability for:

- the proper use of government money: how can the state ensure that voluntary organisations are spending taxpayers' money appropriately?

- correct procedures: how can the state ensure that they follow prescribed procedures in, for example, areas such as child abuse?

- the quality of service they provide: how can the quality of care be monitored and controlled in, for example, voluntary children's homes?

Leat concludes that '[these] problems are likely to increase if a policy of pluralism and closer relationships between the voluntary and statutory sectors are pursued.' By 'pluralism', Leat is referring to the concept of provision through the mixed economy of welfare. The shift to the contracting of services is, in part, designed to force the voluntary sector to be more directly accountable to the government, because contracting involves setting tight specifications and monitoring and inspection procedures. As Davis (1993) shows, however, the process of establishing effective inspection procedures for community care services is highly complex and many issues relating to accountability still remain to be resolved. Nevertheless, the more the priorities and approaches of voluntary organisations are determined by commissioning agencies such as local authorities and health authorities, the less accountable they can be to the groups they represent and to the public which supports them financially and through voluntary effort.

The distribution of voluntary services

A further problem in relying on the voluntary sector to provide a high quality service is the importance of ensuring adequate coverage and uniform distribution. Johnson (1990) cites a number of studies which show that voluntary provision is typically uneven, both geographically and between client groups. Geographical or territorial distribution tends to be related to the socio-economic character of the locality, with middle-class areas generally supporting a higher level of voluntary provision and rural areas often losing out. Data from the Central Statistical Office (1993a) show that people from professional backgrounds are likely to have more time for voluntary work than those in manual occupations and that the highest participation rates are largely in the more affluent South East and South West of England. This may lead to situations where there is an inverse relationship between voluntary provision and need; in other words, areas with less need may actually receive a higher level of provision. As Brenton (1985) concluded in his study of the voluntary sector in Britain, 'Voluntary organisations are thinly and unevenly distributed. Where the need is greatest, they do not exist.'

Some client groups also receive a higher level of support than others, with public sympathy for children and people who are physically disabled being reflected in substantial charitable support, whilst organisations working with groups such as single homeless people, people with learning difficulties and alcohol or drug abusers struggling to attain public support. In addition, people with similar needs may not be equally well-served since voluntary organisations often concentrate their resources on specific groups of people, such as war veterans. This leads Johnson (1990) to conclude that uneven and incomplete coverage leads to overlapping, duplication and waste in some spheres of activity and gaps and shortages in others.

Professionals and volunteers

An important question to be considered in relation to increased reliance on the voluntary sector concerns the boundaries between professional and lay roles in care-giving. The majority of voluntary organisations have been founded in response to needs that have not been met by the statutory sector and they have led the way in pursuing equal opportunity and pioneering new ways of delivering services. Furthermore, the rapid growth of self-help and self-advocacy schemes in which people with common needs or interests support each other has, in large measure, arisen because many service users have found that the services, advice or support they are offered are shaped by the values and beliefs of professional workers rather than their own individual needs. However, many voluntary organisations now employ large numbers of paid professional staff, such as social workers, to undertake key functions and many unpaid trustees volunteer because of their professional interest or experience in working with the organisation's client group. Indeed, in some organisations, voluntary effort is largely confined to the raising of funds: think, for example, of the number of charity shops and fund-raising events run by volunteers. So, even though consumers may be in contact with voluntary organisations, they may in practice be faced with professional workers who have gained their training and experience in the state sector. Brindle (1994c) cites Chris Heginbotham, the chief executive of a mental health NHS trust in London and former director of MIND, who observes that the extent to which professionals can be effective advocates for their client groups is being increasingly questioned:

> 'The trend is for users and carers to want to establish themselves separately. That is happening in mental health particularly, but there is a general desire to be independent of voluntary agencies, to say "We can do it for ourselves". What we will see, I think, is these user groups hiving themselves off from the voluntary organisations, declaring them either paternalistic or too broad to represent their interests. Then the squeeze will really come on these organisations to decide what they want to do – whether they want to be service providers or not.'

A further issue concerning the roles of paid workers and volunteers within voluntary organisations relates to standards. On the one hand, the idealism and altruism associated with voluntarism is one of the greatest strengths of the voluntary sector, particularly where volunteers have similar personal experience to clients that gives them particular insights and empathy for their needs and how they might best be met. On the other hand, voluntary organisations have a responsibility to those who support them, whether government or the general public, to be professional in the way they operate. As Richard Fries (1994), the chief charity commissioner points out 'It is no good having impeccable charitable objects if goodwill is not translated into effective action.' While many aspects of voluntary work do not require training, it is arguable that those who work directly with clients on a voluntary basis should receive sufficient training to enable them to work to agreed standards. Indeed, some contract specifications may include the requirement that volunteers are trained for the tasks they will perform. This, in turn, may create tensions between paid professional and unpaid voluntary workers because of concerns about the exploitation of volunteers or their use as a source of cheap or free labour which may undermine the jobs of paid workers.

Prior to its abolition by the government in 1986, the Greater London Council pursued a policy of supporting the voluntary sector and developed a series of guidelines for policy and practice on volunteers in organisations which it funded. This policy attempted to deal with the difficult political and social issues surrounding volunteering, including the respective roles of volunteers and salaried workers, the importance of guaranteeing standards of service and the need both to promote equal opportunities for volunteers in training and employment and to prevent their exploitation. Although produced a decade ago, it remains interesting because it illustrates the need to protect the interests of all involved in voluntary action – clients, volunteers and paid staff.

ACTIVITY 29 — ALLOW 15 MINUTES

Read *Resource 8*, *The use of volunteers* (GLC, 1985), and note down your ideas about the following questions.

1   Why do you think 1a) is important? Does it imply that the commitment of professional workers only arises as a result of their being paid?

2   1c) refers to the importance of shared similar experiences. Can you suggest any examples of mutual aid groups in your own area?

3   1d) suggests that volunteers themselves should benefit from their involvement. Does this suggest that voluntarism, in this context at least, represents reciprocal altruism?

4   2a) and b) imply that the use of volunteers may make it difficult to guarantee certain standards. Can you suggest why this might be the case?

Commentary

1   For many people who come into contact with voluntary workers, the knowledge that the volunteer is not being paid provides a strong sense of reassurance about that person's level of commitment to them as an individual. They may also feel that 'an ordinary person' will be able to relate to them and empathise more easily. Obviously, many professional staff have a very strong sense of vocation and commitment that drives them towards ever-higher standards and often involves them in work beyond their job description.

2   A quick look at the sections on charitable organisations and social service and welfare organisations in *Yellow Pages* will illustrate the range of voluntary organisations in your area. These may include a number of mutual aid groups where people often find it helpful to talk to others who have had similar experiences, perhaps feeling less reluctant to share their own experiences as a result. Most areas have local Victim Support schemes, branches of Alcoholics Anonymous and local support groups for people who have suffered child abuse, women who have been the victims of domestic violence and people with health problems, such as multiple sclerosis and stroke.

3   Altruism in its purest form exists where donors or volunteers receive nothing for themselves in return for their contribution. Where a volunteer gains some benefit in the form of experience to assist their future career or simply satisfaction from being able to help someone, their voluntary activity is undertaken with the expectation of some form of benefit in return. In other words, it is a form of reciprocal altruism.

4   There may be a problem in relying on volunteers to cover areas where standards need to be guaranteed as voluntary organisations may have difficulties in recruiting suitable people and in providing the required level

of staff training. They may also find it hard to guarantee services because volunteers are bound to them by goodwill rather than by a contractual relationship.

Our discussion of the role of voluntary organisations has shown how some of the principles on which they were founded are increasingly being challenged by their growing role in the mixed economy of welfare. For many, there may be little choice about the direction they will follow in the future. If they enter the 'contract culture', they essentially cease to be voluntary and autonomous and become an arm of the state, however innovative their approaches may continue to be. If they rely on public generosity in an increasingly competitive field, they risk failing to generate sufficient income to be able to support their activities. Government social policy thus plays a key part in determining not only the role of voluntary organisations but also in transforming the very nature of the voluntary sector.

In the next session, we shall consider the impact of social policy on the role of carers and explore some of the potential constraints on an increasing reliance on the informal sector.

Summary

1 The major political parties all acknowledge the contribution that the voluntary sector plays in the provision of welfare services, but disagree on whether their role should be to complement or substitute for statutory provision.

2 The work of the voluntary sector is founded on a tradition of altruism and voluntarism which may be incompatible with a market-led society and may also be threatened by increasing demands on the generosity of the public.

3 A greater role for the voluntary sector has wide-ranging implications in terms of the funding, regulation and distribution of voluntary services.

4 The increasing role of the state in the funding and regulation of the voluntary sector may undermine the very features that have been its strengths. The emphasis on the contracting of services may change the balance between paid and voluntary workers, so that many voluntary organisations become less responsive to the needs of the people they were established to serve.

Before you move on to Session Seven, check that you have achieved the objectives given at the beginning of this session and, if not, review the appropriate sections.

SESSION SEVEN

The 'informal' sector

Introduction

In this session, we shall consider some of the issues raised in Session Three in more detail, focusing on the desirability and feasibility of community care policy which aims to shift the balance away from the state towards the informal sector as the primary provider of care. The term 'informal care' is commonly used to refer to care undertaken by family, friends and neighbours on an informal, unpaid basis and largely in the recipients' own homes. Note, however, that organisations such as the Carers National Association have moved away from the use of the word 'informal' because, to many people, it implies something less important than 'formal', paid, professional care. Here, we shall examine the contribution of care in this sector to the overall provision of welfare in the UK and look at who actually does the caring within the family. We shall then consider some of the implications of this shift from care *in* the community to care *by* the community for the needs of carers themselves.

Session objectives

When you have completed this session, you should be able to:

- identify the main categories of task undertaken by carers

- discuss the advantages and disadvantages of informal and institutional care

- discuss the significance of the gender of carers in determining the level of support provided

- recognise potential constraints on the expansion of the informal sector.

'Informal care'

The foreword to Dalley's *Ideologies of Caring* (1988) outlines some of the very difficult and very important questions that arise in relation to the role of the informal sector:

> 'Where does the responsibility for providing care for dependent people lie? How can the services be offered in ways which do not rely on women to do the unpaid work of caring for members of their own family, or upon the equally sexist assumption that paid jobs which assist the care of dependent people will always be done by women and for very low pay?'

Any discussion about the contribution of informal care must be placed in the context of the increasing emphasis on the transfer of resources and responsibilities away from residential and institutional care in favour of care in the community, particularly since the implementation of the NHS and Community Care Act 1990. The first activity in this session encourages you to think about some of the difficult decisions facing families in relation to caring for dependents.

ACTIVITY 30   ALLOW 20 MINUTES

Read the following case study from Garrett (1990) and then make a list of points which would need to be considered before a decision could be made about Agnes' care.

The Waltons

The Waltons are a couple in their late thirties, living in a three-bedroomed terraced house in a small town, thirty miles away from David's widowed mother, Agnes, who is now aged 73. They have three children: twin boys of 13 and a daughter aged 10. David has a clerical job in the local council offices and Margaret works part-time as a hairdresser.

Agnes has recently suffered a stroke. She is now able to walk with a frame and, despite occasional urinary incontinence, it is felt that she is well enough to leave hospital, although she should not live alone in her council house as she has difficulties with stairs. Her only other child is a single son, Steve, who works as a sales representative for a food company and lives ninety miles away. The grandchildren are very fond of Agnes and David always got on well with both of his parents. He is anxious to bring his mother to live with his family.

Commentary

The first consideration would be Agnes' feelings about the situation. Does she want to live thirty miles away from her old home and friends, with a young, boisterous family? Getting on well during periodic visits is a different thing entirely from living harmoniously together for 365 days a year. Are there alternatives which she would prefer, such as residential care nearer her home?

Of equal concern would be Margaret's feelings. What if she does not get on with Agnes and finds the process of caring distasteful? The bulk of the caring commitment would fall on her, despite the fact that Agnes is not *her* mother. To care for Agnes, Margaret would almost certainly have to give up her job which would have financial implications for the family as well as social implications for her. How would it affect her relationship with David?

Obviously there would be practical considerations, too. Some rearrangement would be needed to accommodate three children and three adults in a three-bedroomed house, with Agnes unable to manage the stairs. One of the downstairs rooms would have to be converted into a bedroom for her, with improvised toilet and washing facilities. How much of her own furniture and how many of her personal belongings would she be able to bring with her? The arrangement would obviously restrict the space available to the rest of the family, at a time when rapidly growing children would normally require more space.

What outside support would Margaret and David be able to get to look after Agnes? Her friends would be thirty miles away and visiting would prove difficult. Is there adequate public transport? What support would the family get through the social services department and from their local health centre? Would day-care provision be available? Some thought would also need to be given to possible weekend and holiday breaks, both for Agnes and for the family. Would Steve be prepared to come to stay and look after Agnes while the others go away or have her to stay at his flat?

These are just some of the considerations that would have to be taken into account before a decision could be made about Agnes' future. In reality, of course, they are not as straightforward as they appear on the surface. Mixed up in them would be all the anxieties about relationships that are common within families, particularly because of the demands that would be made on Margaret and feelings of protectiveness towards the children as well as to Agnes. Both David and Margaret might feel guilt about possibly letting Agnes down as well as being concerned about Margaret's parents who might also suffer as a result of her being tied to the house and having little space for visitors. And, if it seems that the family has a real choice about where Agnes should live, the practical reality may be that there are currently no places for residential or respite care available in any homes in a suitable location.

The important contribution of the informal sector has been recognised for some time. Even a decade ago, the Family Policy Studies Centre (FPSC) estimated that the value of informal care ranged from £15 to £24 billion per year (Parker, 1985), although estimates of this kind are very difficult to make with any accuracy as the defining feature of this sector is its largely hidden nature. The FPSC figure was based on a notional rate of payment of £4 per hour, irrespective of the level of care provided, but it took no account of additional expenditure for requirements such as travel or adaptations to the home or of the opportunity costs in terms of the careers and wages that might be foregone by carers. Neither did it take account of the costs of any child care that might be needed to enable carers to attend to the needs of (non-child) dependents. The FPSC figure is useful, however, if only to illustrate the contribution of the informal sector in relation to total government expenditure on social services which, in 1992, amounted to £6.56 billion (Central Statistical Office, 1994b).

What kinds of functions does 'informal' care involve? The following activity asks you to consider the type of support that a dependent person may require.

ACTIVITY 31 — ALLOW 10 MINUTES

Think about any families whom you know personally or professionally in which one or more people are dependent on others to provide care. They may be people who are elderly or disabled or who have mental health problems or learning difficulties. Sketch out two brief case studies and note down the various kinds of support required by each dependent person.

Commentary

You may have listed such tasks as cleaning, laundry, shopping, cooking, bathing, continence care, collecting pensions or allowances, providing emotional support and companionship, and organising outings, but the kinds of support required by each person will obviously depend on their individual needs and circumstances. In their study of informal care, Willmott and Thomas (1984) identified the following five categories of task:

1 **Personal care**: including washing, bathing, dressing and toileting and general attention to bodily needs and comforts.

2 **Domestic care**: including cooking, cleaning and laundering.

3 **Auxiliary care**: including less onerous tasks such as baby-sitting, child-minding, shopping, transport, odd-jobbing, gardening, borrowing and lending.

4 **Social support**: including visiting and companionship.

5 **Surveillance**: essentially keeping an eye on vulnerable people.

These distinctions are important as the nature of the task is often linked to the relationship of the carer, as we shall see later in this session.

Institutional care

As we have already seen, one of the great benefits of informal care – at least to the government – is that it is a cheap option. A second, powerful argument for the expansion of the informal sector is that families and other carers can provide a higher quality of care and that dependent people, be they elderly, disabled or children, have a greater degree of autonomy in informal care settings. Part of this concern reflects a very negative image of residential or institutional care in the UK which is typically associated with all institutions, including residential care homes, nursing homes and psychogeriatric units, children's homes, mental hospitals and prisons.

ACTIVITY 32

Think about a residential home or institution that you know or talk to someone such as an older relative who has experience of institutional care, perhaps in a nursing home or residential care home. What do you think are some of the advantages and disadvantages of institutional care as far its residents are concerned?

Commentary

From the perspective of its residents, an institutional setting is likely to be judged on the extent to which it meets their individual needs. It may offer specialist, professional care that could not be provided in the home, resulting in a sense of reassurance and security, particularly for those who have a high level of dependency. Residents are freed from the pressures of daily life, such as shopping and cleaning, and may have greater opportunities for social interaction and companionship. On the other hand, the enforced separation from all that is familiar, the lack of control over their environment, their daily routine and their food, the potential loss of privacy and dignity and prolonged periods of isolation and boredom may all combine to make institutional care a profoundly depressing experience, particularly for those who are aware they are unlikely ever to return home to be near their family, friends and neighbours.

For many people, dissatisfaction with residential care stems from frustration about their own level of dependency. Nevertheless, the way in which care is provided obviously makes a significant difference to the quality of life for residents. You may know of institutions that are lively places offering a wide range of activities and are run in a way that permits every element of flexibility and autonomy possible, bearing in mind the needs of the client group. As Garrett (1990) found, there can be a considerable degree of active participation by residents in the running of their homes:

> 'Many homes now have residents' committees which discuss issues of interest and importance to the people living there, and which make decisions on a whole variety of topics – from which part of the lounge should be a no-smoking area, to where to go for a spring outing.'

Indeed, as Fitzpatrick and Taylor (1994a; 1994b) found in their study to evaluate care from the patient perspective, service users may have very different ideas from professional carers and members of their families about what makes an institutional setting a good place to be. In their work to elicit the criteria by which patients in long-stay wards for elderly people judge a good service, they found that the personal attributes of professional carers were most valued but that patients also attached particularly high importance to visitors. Seven out of the 13 top ranked criteria concerned the organisational aspects of their care: having a choice and variety in the food offered, having company and the chance to make friends, eating at a table, church services, having a permanent place in the ward and not being moved, visiting times and concert parties. Only two criteria related to the management of care for the individual: privacy and dignity and knowing what their tablets were for. When relatives and nurses were similarly asked to identify the essential requirements for a good service for elderly patients in long-term hospital care, however, they were successful in identifying only one third of the criteria that the patients themselves had selected, as shown in *Figure 17*. Significantly, Fitzpatrick and Taylor found that the patients did not perceive themselves as being 'customers' of the health service with any possibility of determining their living conditions, finding that they tended to associate choice with the private sector, or rather a lack of choice with the statutory sector. In the words of one patient, 'There are plenty of homes round here. There are over a dozen which you can pick and choose for anyone who really wants to get into a place where they've got private rooms, who can make their tea whenever it suits them ... but you've got to go into a private home ... this is an NHS hospital.'

In practice, the common negative view of residential care tends to tar all forms of institution with the same brush, despite the variations that exist between different establishments. While one of the aims of community care is to avoid people

Table 1. The top 13 ranked criteria for a good service as ranked by patients in long-stay wards for elderly people.

Patients' criteria	Score
Nurses attentive/cheerful/listen	82
Visitors	75
Company/chance to make friends	15
Cleanliness of wards	15
Church services	12
Knowing what your tablets are for	38
Privacy/dignity	37
Permanent place in the ward	36
Eating at a table	35
Occupational therapy	29
Food – variety and choice	28
Visiting times	28
Concert parties	26

Table 2. The top 13 ranked criteria for a good service as ranked by relatives of patients in long-stay wards for elderly people

Relatives' criteria	Score
Nurses attentive/cheerful/listen	53
Privacy/dignity	52
Cleanliness of wards	49
Physiotherapy	49
Safe/appropriate aids	31
More untrained carers	30
Continuity of care/same staff	30
Food - choice and variety	29
Carers with a vocation	28
Toileting	24
Own choice of clothes and toiletries	23
Continued medical treatment	21
Grooming	21

Table 3. The top 13 ranked criteria for a good service as ranked by nurses of patients in long-stay wards for elderly people

Nurses' criteria	Score
Nurses attentive/cheerful/listen	71
Food - choice and variety	49
Own clothes and toiletries	49
Decor and furnishing	43
Personalised care	40
Visitors	39
Privacy/dignity	37
Personal belongings	35
Toilet facilities	31
Outside information	23
TV/radio/books	22
Warmth and lighting	20
Safe/appropriate aids	20

Figure 17: The top 13 ranked criteria for a good service as ranked by patients, relatives and nurses in long-stay wards for elderly people (Fitzpatrick and Taylor, 1994a)

being forced into institutional care unnecessarily, much of the impetus for the expansion of informal care has come from critiques of institutionalisation, particularly the work of Townsend (1962) and Goffman (1968) which characterised the 'total institution' as being dehumanising and resistant to change. Such stereotypes have led to the popular belief that all institutional care is inherently inferior in terms of the standards of care offered and that it is always more costly.

Long before the implementation of the NHS and Community Care Act 1990, Jones and Fowles (1983) observed that the American notion of deinstitutionalisation was providing a major impetus to initiatives in the UK that were increasingly aimed at preventing the entry of people to institutions and emptying existing institutions in favour of care in the community. Tizard (1975) had already criticised calls for the wholesale abandonment of institutional care and argued that much of the earlier research, such as that by Townsend and Goffman, was based on individual case studies and should not be seen as representative of institutional care *per se*. He highlighted the varieties of residential experience and suggested the importance of taking account of the differences between institutions in terms of their regimes and recruitment as well as in the degree of autonomy for occupants and variations in staff attitudes and behaviour which, he suggested, may reflect levels of pay and staff training.

Opposition to the concept of institutional provision and the consequent pressure for the expansion of informal care often still seems to rest on stereotypical notions of large, monolithic and segregative Victorian-style institutions that bear little resemblance to many modern residential units. However, the belief that all institutions are 'bad' and that family care is always 'good' is increasingly being challenged by evidence on the extent of abuse against elderly people, child abuse and domestic violence that takes place within the family (Abbott and Wallace, 1990).

With the closure of many long-stay wards and mental hospitals, the general perception is that institutional care is declining overall, even though this is not the case as far as some groups are concerned. Throughout the 1980s and early 1990s, for example, there was a steady increase in the number of elderly people in residential accommodation, as shown in *Figure 18*, partly as a result of the changing age-structure of the population as well as the expansion of the private

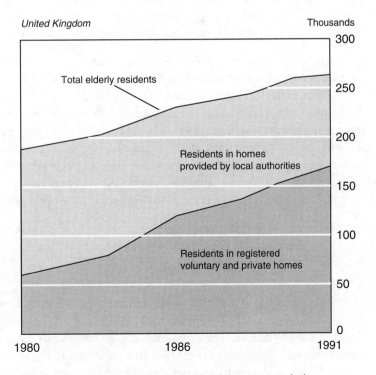

Figure 18: Elderly people in residential accommodation
(Source: Central Statistical Office, 1993a)

sector in the provision of residential care. As we saw in Session Five, this explosion in institutional provision is largely financed and regulated by the state through social services and social work departments and health authorities. In assessing the implications of deinstitutionalisation, therefore, it is important to remember that the role of the state is changing, but not necessarily declining.

We have seen how the impetus for the expansion of the informal sector has come from two main directions. First, it is seen as being cheaper and this is particularly important during a period of tight control on public expenditure. Second, it is considered to provide higher quality of care for dependents. There is obviously a strong argument for increasing the range of options open to people who cannot live independently and, for many, care in their own home or that of their family is certainly the preferred option. On the other hand, many people whose capacity for self-care is limited do not wish to live with their family, not least because this may undermine their own independence and they fear becoming a burden. It is also important to consider the implications of the argument about choice and the quality of care from the perspective of the carer – one person's free choice may mean the denial of choice for another. In order to explore this issue in more detail, we need to look at who actually does the bulk of the caring within the family.

Who does the caring?

In 1985, 6 million people were carers. By 1990, the General Household Survey (Office of Population Censures and Surveys, 1992) showed that this figure had risen to 6.8 million people – 15% of the population compared with 14% in 1985. Of these, 24% were aged 45–64, compared with 8% of those aged 16–29, 15% of those aged 30–44 and 15% of those aged 65 or over, many of whom reported that they themselves had some form of long-standing illness. More than 24% were spending more than 20 hours a week caring, while 11% were devoting more than 50 hours a week to their caring role. Most carers look after elderly people; in 1990, 79% of those cared for were over 65 and 20% were 85 or over, an increase of 5% since 1985 (Carers National Association, 1994a).

While popular belief suggests that the vast majority of carers are women, 13% of men said they were carers (2.9 million) and 17% of women (3.9 million) said they were carers. However, the Equal Opportunities Commission (1984) compared the contributions of men and women in the care of elderly dependent people and found that women were much more likely to take responsibility for personal and domestic care duties, such as washing. The contribution of male family members, whilst substantially less than that of women, was largely restricted to Willmott and Thomas's (1984) category of 'auxiliary care'. Nissell and Bonnerjea (1982) similarly found that husbands rarely gave help to their wives with the care of the

dependent relative living with them, even when the wife was also employed. As Parker (1985) argued, in her review of research on informal care, to talk about community or family care is to disguise reality:

> 'In fact ... "care by the community" almost always means care by family members with little support from others in the "community". Further, care by family members almost always means care by female members with little support from other relatives. It appears that "shared care" is uncommon; once one person has been identified as the main carer, other relatives withdraw.'

Typically, care is provided by the wife, daughter or daughter-in-law, with very little support from other family members. In addition, where the state actually provides services such as home helps, meals-on-wheels or day-centre places to support carers in their work, evidence from the Equal Opportunities Commission (EOC) suggests that it is male carers who are more likely to be allocated the services, as shown in *Figure 19*.

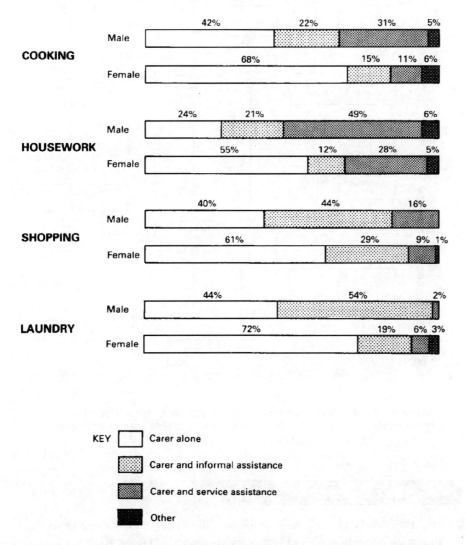

Figure 19: Receipt of informal and service assistance with domestic care and personal care tasks by sex of carer (Source: Equal Opportunities Commission, 1984)

In addition, as *Figure 20* shows, the EOC found that government-funded support services tend to become involved in supporting female carers at a much later stage in the caring process than for male carers. This is particularly evident in relation to the provision of service support for non-spouse carers living with an elderly person. As you can see, when the non-spouse living with an elderly person is female there is typically no home help or meals-on-wheels provision, community nursing support is received slightly later in the process and intermittent day care tends to be introduced at the point of dependency when an elderly person living with a male non-spouse would have been offered long-stay residential care. Why do you think these differences in service allocation exist?

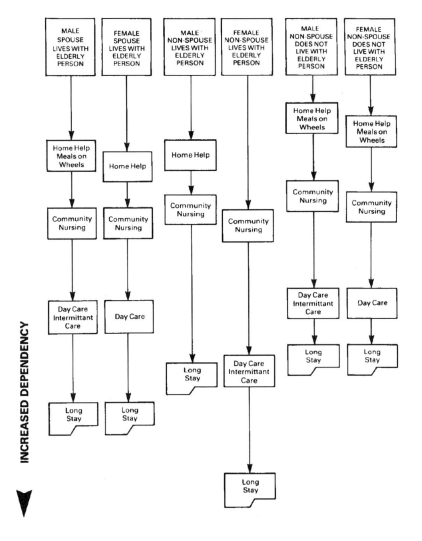

Figure 20: Schematic representation of patterns of service support by carer's relationship with elderly person, and degree of elderly person's dependency (Source: Equal Opportunities Commission, 1984)

ACTIVITY 33   ALLOW **10** MINUTES

List at least three possible reasons for the differences in the pattern of service allocation between male and female carers shown in *Figure 20*.

Commentary

It could be argued that male carers have less skill and experience in areas of domestic work than women and, in particular, may have little experience of cooking or cleaning. Additionally, where personal tasks are required, such as assistance with bathing, it may be considered inappropriate for a male relative to assist, particularly where the dependent person is female. Where the carer is male and in full-time work, he is more likely to be supported by service providers on the grounds that he is the bread-winner and needs to be enabled to continue in this role. The same argument is less likely to be applied to women, particularly if they are married. It is generally presumed in such cases that the woman can give up work without upsetting the household budget too seriously. Of course, in many cases such assumptions are ill-founded and, as Abbott and Wallace (1990) have demonstrated, fail to recognise the importance of women's incomes to the family budget.

Dalley (1988) refers to the dominance of Conservative thinking about the role of the family, and of women within the family, in the structuring of the 'whole social organisation of daily living and thus directly [in] producing the forms of caring'. Community care, she argues, has been actively promoted by right-wing sections of the Conservative Party not only as a way of saving on the heavy costs of institutional care, but also as the most appropriate and natural form of care for the dependent person. This view fits in neatly with the residualist approach to welfare that we discussed in Session One, whereby the family is seen as the primary source of care with the role of the statutory sector being to provide care only when that source has broken down in some way.

Dalley also makes an important distinction between caring *for* people and caring *about* people, a distinction that many feminists have raised as a defence against the accusation that they do not care as 'normal' women should. If a woman is unable or does not want to take on the role of unpaid carer, it is assumed that she is 'unnatural' or selfish and does not care. Dalley suggests that Conservative thinking about the family and its role in society fuses these two aspects of caring for women so that, in order to demonstrate genuine 'care', they have to care about and also to care for dependent people. Men, on the other hand, are able to demonstrate that they care about dependent family members by taking financial responsibility for them, perhaps by providing the family home or buying in services, but they are not expected to care for their personal and domestic needs to the same extent. As we have seen, they are not generally expected to do the hands-on caring such as toileting or bathing, or to give up their work role to care for dependents on a full-time basis. As Dalley concludes:

> 'Whenever policy documents talk about the responsibility, willingness and the duty of families to provide care – and [the government White Paper] *Growing Older* (DHSS, 1981) is a good example – the substance of these statements is that they mean *women* will do the physical and emotional providing for, whilst men should underwrite this effort financially.'

While commentators such as Dalley challenge the desirability of an increasing reliance on unpaid women carers from an equal opportunities perspective, it is also important to consider the extent to which it will actually be feasible, given the changing demographic and social factors that need to be taken into account. In common with most of Western Europe, the UK has an ageing population. At the same time, the size of family units is becoming smaller, the average household having fallen from just over three people in 1961 to 2.5 people in 1991. The reduction in the size of family units, coupled with the increase in the number and proportion of elderly members of the population, means that far fewer women will be available to look after increasing numbers of dependent people.

Another factor that has implications for community care is the impact of geographic mobility, with many potential carers now living considerable distances from their elderly parents as employment policies and economic pressures encourage people to move in order to find work. At the same time, there has been a substantial increase in labour force participation rates amongst women. Johnson (1990) cites data demonstrating an increase of 74% in the number of economically active women in the period 1950–1980 compared to an increase of 25% for men. By 1992, 53% of women of working age were working either full-time or part-time, although the proportion was around 70% for women under the age of 55 (Central Statistical Office, 1994a). In 1982, the EOC found that the majority of carers were women under retirement age, some of whom are likely to have given up paid employment in order to take on the role of carer. However, as Finch and Groves (1983) have commented, there is a tendency to ignore the issue of 'whether women will continue to accept their cultural designation as carers, or whether they will explicitly reject it, in ideology and in practice, in increasing numbers.' In other words, for how long will women be prepared – or able – to give up the financial and social benefits that come with working in order to play a caring role? Furthermore, widespread changes in family structures such as the increase in lone-parenting raise questions about individuals' responsibilities and obligations towards different categories of kin. The divorce rate doubled between 1971 and 1991, for example, and for every two marriages in Britain in 1991, there was one divorce (Central Statistical Office, 1994a). What obligations does a woman have towards an ex-mother-in-law?

Young carers

A particular area of concern is the growing number of young carers of school age and below. In 1993, the Carers National Association (CNA) estimated that well over 10,000 children act as primary carers nationwide. Commonly, they are from lone-parent families in which the parent develops a disabling illness, although there is also an unknown number living with an elderly grandparent or providing emotional stability in a family which experiences mental distress, and older children are often needed to help out with a disabled sibling. As the CNA warns, where 'helping out' becomes a responsibility rather than simply a normal part of family life, there can be serious effects on the child's personal and educational development.

> 'As well as the physical side of caring – washing, dressing and feeding – there is evidence that emotional pressures can lead to difficulties in forming social relationships. Poor school attendance is common; but so too is a quiet denial of problems through fear and loyalty. In these respects, young carers have more in common with other "children in need" than with adult carers. In the past, the focus has been the needs of the disabled member of the family. Many young people are losing out on their childhood and youth in this way.'

The Children Act 1989 and the NHS and Community Care Act 1990 should provide a stronger and more flexible legislative framework for addressing the needs of young carers, but the CNA stresses that unless attitudes and practice change significantly, the needs of children who are carers will continue to be ignored. It emphasises the need for statutory and voluntary agencies to work together to provide an integrated range of services by:

- including provision for young carers when planning future services and looking at innovative approaches such as advocacy and befriending

- revising training programmes to ensure a sensitive and consistent response from staff

- making home care services more accessible and appropriate to children

- addressing the additional stigma that can face children of people with mental illness, AIDS, genetic disorders or difficulties with substance abuse

- examining their approach to ethnic minority families where children often act as interpreters.

The CNA also points out the societal pressure on disabled parents themselves to be 'model parents', citing one mother who found that 'Because I use a wheelchair, I can't get to the children's appointments. If I miss appointments, they tell me I'm not caring. Then they start talking about care proceedings.' Scarce resources and a lack of information add to the pressure they face and families who fear that their children will be taken into care are often unwilling to let professional workers know they need help, thus increasing the demands on young carers even further.

Who cares for the carers?

Finch and Groves (1983) refer to the reality of community care as a 'double equation' in that 'in practice community care equals care by the family, and in practice care by the family equals care by women.' Although the Conservative Party claims wide public support for an increased role for the informal sector, this may in fact be more a reflection of its own beliefs than a true reflection of society's views. A survey by West (1984) on public attitudes towards family responsibilities concluded that:

> 'In the sample as a whole the idea of family care alone receives support from only a minority of respondents...The public as a whole are strongly supportive of professional and service involvement in the care of dependent persons.'

A major reason why the public may not be as committed to care in the community as the government would wish is that, as Parker (1985) emphasises, the full cost of informal care has to take into account the cost to women in terms of their employment opportunities, earnings potential, increased expenditure, physical illness and disability, and emotional stress. While many carers gladly assume responsibility for the care of a dependent person, the strain on them is often considerable. The physical and psychological costs of caring have been highlighted in a number of studies cited by Pollock (1994), including a survey by the Carers National Association (Pitkeathley, 1992) which showed that two thirds of the respondents were over 55 years of age, nearly half were caring for someone aged 75 or over and two thirds of them felt their own health had suffered as a result of their caring duties. For many carers, the physical and emotional demands, a sense of social isolation and a feeling of being undervalued result in severe stress and fatigue that not only affects their own health but also the quality of the care that they can give.

Clearly, many people want to play an active role in supporting and looking after their dependents but, in order to assess whether the policy of increasing reliance on the informal sector is both viable and just, we need to consider how the state can play a more active role in facilitating the expansion of this sector without putting carers under excessive pressure.

ACTIVITY 34   ALLOW 15 MINUTES

What do you think are the main areas of support that carers need from professional agencies? You may find it helpful to talk to a relative or a friend who is a carer to find out the aspects of care that they find most demanding.

Commentary

In their research study on informal care, Nolan and Grant (1989) found that the needs of carers are all too often overlooked. According to them, 'A failure adequately to conceptualise the needs of carers has, in the past, resulted in interventions often being inappropriate, irrelevant or unavailable.' They identified four key areas of deficiency associated with carers' interactions with professional agencies:

- a lack of information about access to services

- a lack of skills training, such as in being taught how to lift properly

- a lack of emotional support

- a lack of regular respite care for their dependents.

A survey conducted by the Carers National Association through a consumer magazine (reported in *Nursing Times*, 1993), supported their conclusions. Half of the carers who responded wanted a cheaper and better respite service, saying it was the only way to get some 'normality' into their lives. They also identified a need for special equipment, financial help and counselling, calling for a network of local support groups or a free counselling service to help them emotionally. One in five said they needed greater recognition of their role and 16% said they were treated as second-class citizens or were talked down to.

Resource 9, Carers Code: Eight key principles for health and social care providers was developed by the Carers National Association (1994b) in collaboration with local authorities and the support of the Association of Directors of Social Services. It provides an important guide for professional workers on ways in which they can ensure that the needs of carers, as well as those for whom they care, are fully taken into account when planning and delivering services. It underlines the importance of providing support services before a crisis occurs, thereby enabling carers to continue their caring role and preventing unnecessary hospitalisation or residential care.

The government White Paper, *Caring for People* (Department of Health, 1989b) recognised that carers not only have needs, but that they have equal needs to services and support as those for whom they care. Indeed, it identified services that respond flexibly and sensitively to the needs of individuals and their carers as the key component of community care and the second of the six key objectives of service delivery specified the aim 'to ensure that service providers make practical support for carers a high priority'.

'While this White Paper focuses largely on the role of statutory and independent bodies in the provision of community care services, the reality is that most care is provided by family, friends and neighbours. The majority of carers take on these responsibilities willingly, but the government recognises that many need help to be able to manage what can become a heavy burden. Their lives could be made much easier if the right support is there at the right time, and a key responsibility of the statutory service providers should be to do all they can to assist and support carers. Helping carers to maintain their valuable contribution to the spectrum of care is both right and a sound investment. Help may take the form of providing advice and support as well as practical services such as day, domiciliary and respite care.'

Despite government commitment to improve support for carers, however, there remains a large shortfall in the kind and level of services required to meet their needs and facilitate the development of effective community care. In practice, resources tend to be targeted on individuals who are unsupported and, as Pitkeathley (1991) comments, 'For too long the presence of a carer in the household has been the signal for service providers to breathe a sigh of relief and think that they do not need to worry about the particular problem.' A year after the implementation of the community care reforms in April 1993, a survey conducted for the Carers National Association (Warner, 1994) found that 74% of the people caring for an elderly or disabled relative or friend said that there had been no assessment of the needs of the person they care for, let alone of their needs as carers. 27% did not even realise that local authority social service departments have assumed responsibility for assessing needs and arranging services. Since the survey was conducted among carers in touch with some form of voluntary group, the association fears that other 'hidden' carers would know even less about community care. As Warner observed, 'The jury is still out on whether the community care changes will improve the lot of carers. On the evidence of this preliminary study, carers are distinctly underwhelmed.'

Summary

1   The major impetus for the expansion of the informal sector stems from two main factors:

- anticipated savings in public expenditure through a greater reliance on unpaid family labour for the provision of care

- the view that informal carers provide a personal service that is generally superior in quality to that provided in institutional care.

2   The majority of carers are women who generally receive little assistance from other family members in personal and domestic care tasks, although the number of male carers and young carers is growing. Women invariably receive less support from the statutory sector, and at a later stage, than male carers.

3   Any further proposed expansion in the role of the informal sector may be constrained by:

- demographic changes that will alter the ratio of potential care-givers to dependents

- increasing geographic mobility which will restrict the availability of informal care within the community

- increased participation by women in the labour market, which limits the time available for them to undertake unpaid caring

- changes in family structure.

4   Despite the advantages of increased reliance on informal care, many carers do not receive a sufficient level of support. This places an immense strain on them and their families which, in turn, may have serious implications for the quality of care that they are able to provide.

Before you move on to Session Eight, check that you have achieved the objectives given at the beginning of this session and, if not, review the appropriate sections.

SESSION EIGHT

Social policy and concepts of need

Introduction

In this final session, we return to the concept of need. You will recall from your work on Session One that meeting need is generally accepted to be one of the main functions of social policy. Here, we shall look more closely at what is meant by the term 'need' and consider how the way in which it is defined helps to determine the nature of the response. In particular, we shall focus on need in relation to a specific group of people – people with disabilities – in order to show how the relevance and effectiveness of welfare provision is, to some extent, dependent on who defines the 'need' that services are designed to meet. This should help to illustrate how the outcomes of social policy are shaped not only by policy makers but also by those who are responsible for its implementation, whether in the statutory, private, voluntary or informal sectors.

Session objectives

When you have completed this session, you should be able to:

- discuss need as a relative concept

- suggest why the way in which needs are defined has important implications for social policy

- discuss how the definitions of need adopted by health and social care professionals can affect the experiences of those for whom they care.

Poverty and need

Much of the literature on social policy talks in terms of 'poverty' and 'needs'. Essentially, both poverty and need are relative concepts in Western societies. 'Absolute poverty' typically refers to subsistence conditions; for a person, household or area to be defined as being in absolute poverty, they would have to lack basic shelter, food, water and clothing. It is generally held that such poverty has been largely eradicated in Britain, although there is increasing evidence that it still exists. Kempson, Bryson and Rowlingson (1994), for example, found that more than half the mothers in the low-income families they surveyed in five inner-city areas regularly go without food to protect their children from poverty.

Relative poverty is 'relative' to the extent that it assumes the existence of some societal norm. It reflects the assumptions of ordinary people or of dominant groups within that society, such as politicians or professionals, about culturally and socially acceptable standards of living. The contention is not that people are 'poor' *per se*, but that they are poor in relation to prevailing living standards. As the influential report *Faith in the City*, published in 1985 by the General Synod of the Church of England, concluded:

> 'Poverty is not only about shortage of money. It is about rights and relationships; about how people are treated and how they regard themselves; about powerlessness, exclusion and loss of dignity. Yet the lack of an adequate income is at its heart.'

The concept of relative poverty is more complex than that of absolute poverty and is based on the contention that it is possible to determine, within any particular society, a poverty line or a level of means below which a person is regarded as being poor. Once this poverty line has been established, families or individuals with an income or means, including savings, falling below that level are defined as suffering from relative poverty. For the purposes of policy development, such as determining the level at which welfare benefits or services will be provided, therefore, it is necessary to arrive at a working definition of poverty and to identify whether there is a social consensus – that is, whether the public generally agrees – on what constitutes an acceptable standard of living or quality of life. The problem is one of deciding how to identify what an acceptable standard is.

ACTIVITY 35   ALLOW 10 MINUTES

Imagine that you are planning to undertake some research on poverty in the UK and want to find out how many people could be defined as poor. In order to obtain this information, you would need to devise some method of establishing what your poverty line is going to be. How would you go about setting a poverty line? Who would you talk to and what would you ask them?

Commentary

In order to set a poverty line, you would obviously need to gather information from a variety of sources, including statistical data on income and expenditure, unemployment, social security, housing and ill-health. You would need to talk to specialists in the welfare services such as social workers, Citizens Advice Bureaux workers and debt counsellors who work on a daily basis with people who are poor. In order to reflect the social consensus at a particular point in time, you would need to find out the level of means that the average person in the street considers to be necessary in order to keep a family out of poverty. You would also need to look at the findings of research studies on social policy and perhaps to talk to researchers who, you may feel, might offer the most objective and informed view.

Your choice of people to talk to would have important implications for the number of people defined as poor since the perceptions of various groups are likely to differ. Professionals who have limited personal experience of poverty, for example, might define it in a way that reflects their own values rather than those of members of society who would consider themselves to be poor. They may, for instance, feel that an indoor toilet is a basic requirement when some elderly people who have lived all their lives with an outdoor lavatory may feel affronted at the suggestion that this would classify them as being poor. Similarly, they might exclude items that some people would consider essential, such as Christmas presents for their children, cigarettes or a video recorder.

It would also be necessary to ensure that you talk to a large enough number of people to ensure a representative view. This would be particularly important if you chose to canvass the opinions of the general public and you would also need to ensure that a large number of people from a range of backgrounds and geographic locations, ages, ethnic groups and across both genders are included.

In 1985, Mack and Lansley attempted to develop an operational definition of poverty based on the values of a cross-section of the public. In particular, they asked two questions:

> Is there a degree of social consensus over what constitutes acceptable minimum standards in Britain today?

> If so, which items are necessary and should, therefore, be affordable by all?

They conducted a survey of 1,174 people aged 18 and over and asked them to indicate which, out of a list of over 35 possible items, they considered to be necessities. From this they constructed the list, shown in *Figure 21,* ranked in order of the importance attached to the items by the respondents.

NECESSITIES OF LIFE

1. Heating
2. Indoor toilet
3. Damp-free home
4. Bath
5. Bed for everyone
6. Public transport
7. Warm waterproof coat
8. Three meals a day for children
9. Self-contained accommodation
10. Two pairs of all-weather shoes
11. Sufficient bedrooms for children
12. Refrigerator
13. Toys for children
14. Carpets
15. Celebrations on special occasions
16. Roast joint once a week
17. Washing machine
18. New, not second-hand clothes
19. Hobby or leisure activity
20. Two hot meals a day (adults)
21. Meat/fish every other day
22. Presents once a year
23. Holiday
24. Leisure equipment for children
25. Garden
26. Television

Figure 21: The necessities of life (Source: Mack and Lansley, 1985)

Using this list, Mack and Lansley were then able to work out how much money a family required in order to be able to afford these items.

The Joseph Rowntree Memorial Trust (1992) later undertook a similar survey of a cross-section of the population, asking them to indicate what they considered to be the basic necessities of life. The research team then used the list obtained from the research to cost two budgets which it called the 'modest but adequate' budget and the 'low-cost' budget. *Figure 22* shows both what the basket of goods includes for each of the budgets and what it does not include. In order to sustain the modest but adequate budget, a typical family of two adults living with two children under 10 would have required an income of £317 a week at 1992 prices. A similar family on a low-cost budget would have required an income of £141 per week – 30% more than they could obtain through income support.

Low Cost Budget		Modest but Adequate Budget	
Examples of items included	**Examples of items excluded**	**Examples of items included**	**Examples of items excluded**
Basic furniture, textiles and hardware	Antiques, handmade or precious household durables	Basic designs, mass manufactured furniture, textiles and hardware	Antiques, handmade or precious household durables
First aid kit and basic medicine	Prescription, dental and sight care charges	Prescription charges, dental care, sight test	Spectacles, private health care
Fridge, washing machine, lawn mower and vacuum cleaner	Freezer, tumble-dryer, shower, electric blankets, microwave, food-mixer	Fridge-freezer, washing machine, microwave, food-mixer, sewing machine	Tumble-dryer, shower, electric blankets
Basic clothing (cheapest prices in C&A)	Second-hand, designer and high fashion clothing	Basic clothing, sensible designs	Second-hand, designer and high fashion clothing
TV, video hire, cassette player, basic camera	Hi-fi, children's TVs, compact discs, camcorders	TV, video hire, basic music system and camera	Children's TVs, compact discs, camcorders
Public transport, children's bikes	Car, adult bikes, caravan, camping equipment	Second-hand 5-year-old car, second-hand adult bicycle, new children's bikes	A second car, caravan, camping equipment, mountain bikes
Clocks, watches	Jewellery	Basic jewellery, watch	Precious jewellery
Haircuts	Cosmetics	Basic cosmetics, haircuts	Perfume, hair perm
	Alcohol/smoking	Alcohol – men 14 units, women 10 units (2/3 HEA safe limit)	Smoking
Day-trip to Blackpool	Annual holiday	One week annual holiday	Holiday abroad
Cinema twice a year, visiting museums and historic buildings about twice a year	Concerts, panto, ballet, or music lessons for children	Walking, swimming, cycling, football, cinema, panto every two years, youth clubs, scouts/guides	Fishing, water sports, horse-riding, creative or educational adult classes, children's ballet/music lessons

Figure 22: Household budgets and living standards
(Source: Joseph Rowntree Foundation, 1992)

Obviously, the income of a household directly affects the pattern of its expenditure and determines whether it has any real choices about how to spend its money. Government data shows, for example, that households with less than £100 of disposable income per week devoted nearly a quarter of their expenditure to food and a further quarter to housing, fuel, light and power in 1992. In contrast, those with over £400 of weekly disposable income devoted only 15% of their total expenditure to food and a further 20% to housing, fuel, light and power (Central Statistical Office, 1994a).

The ability to purchase consumer goods is a valid indicator of poverty. But the issue of money and purchasing power is not simply about the ownership of or access to goods; it reflects a more fundamental question that concerns the level of equality within a society and people's ability to participate in it. In reviewing the subsistence concept – that is, the view that we can define poverty by reference to access to certain minimal social goods necessary for our subsistence – Townsend (1979) arrived at the following definition of poverty based on the relative concept of our ability to participate in 'normal' everyday life:

> 'Individuals can be said to be in poverty when they lack the resources to obtain the types of diet, participate in the activities and have the living conditions and amenities which are customary, or at least widely encouraged or approved, in the societies to which they belong.'

If a family cannot afford a television licence, for instance, they can't watch the latest soap opera. But if the conversation at playtime or in the staff canteen is regularly about that programme, they may be excluded from an important aspect of social interaction within their peer group. Children whose parents cannot afford to give them more than a token present may find it hard to face going to school to be asked by their friends what they got for their birthday. You may remember media reports about the child who became the victim of bullying because she did not have the 'correct' brand of trainers to wear at school and truanted as a result. A health care professional may be reluctant to include in their list of necessary goods the price of a few pints of beer or its equivalent, but that may mean that a person cannot afford to go to the local pub that is the main locus of social activity in that area. While not having access to certain goods may not mean that a person is living in absolute poverty, it may result in a painful and debilitating degree of social stigma resulting in isolation, loneliness and low self-esteem. As we saw in Session Two, research evidence suggests that inequalities in health are not caused simply by the direct physiological impact of poverty and that the social and psychological meanings attached to material differences also have a tangible impact on health and well-being.

Significantly, the Supplementary Benefits Commission (cited in Andrews & Jacobs, 1990) had already reached a similar conclusion in 1978, when its annual report contained the following modest prescription for how any civilised nation ought to treat its citizens.

> 'To keep out of poverty, [claimants] must have an income which enables them to participate in the life of the community. They must be able, for example, to keep themselves reasonably well-fed, and well enough dressed to maintain their self-respect and to attend interviews for jobs with confidence. Their homes must be reasonably warm; their children should not feel ashamed by the quality of their clothing; the family must be able to visit relatives, and give them

> something on their birthdays and at Christmas time; they must be able to read newspapers, and retain their televisions sets and their membership of trade unions and churches. And they must be able to live in a way which ensures, so far as possible, that public officials, doctors, teachers, landlords and others treat them with the courtesy due to every member of the community.'

Thus, a person or household or area is 'poor' if it lacks something that society deems to be a necessity at that point in time. The definition of poverty, then, is not static, but is constantly modified according to:

- changing social attitudes

- prevailing economic circumstances: values may, for instance, change during or after a recession

- shifting political priorities and values, such as different governmental attitudes towards unemployment.

Accordingly, the way in which poverty is defined, together with perceptions of its causes, helps to shape the policy responses that might be considered appropriate. During the 1990s, for example, the concept of a growing 'underclass' has increasingly been accepted on the right of the political spectrum. This term is used to characterise groups of people whose prolonged experience of poverty, unemployment and dependence on welfare benefits is seen to have resulted in their alienation from mainstream society and their failure to share many of its commonly-accepted values. One of the most influential proponents of this view is Murray (1990; 1994), a right-wing American political scientist, who argues that the underclass in Britain is a sub-section of society whose poverty is a consequence of its own 'deplorable behaviour', which is particularly manifested in the growth of illegitimacy and lone parenthood. As Becker (1995) observes:

> 'The rarity of public scenes of mass squalor, and the hidden nature of poverty, have reinforced the "common sense view" that the problem of poverty has now been overtaken by the much more pressing problem of the benefit fraudster and other groups of "non-deserving" poor. This perception, that it is the poor or unscrupulous fraudster – not poverty – that is a cause for concern, has been a consistent theme of government rhetoric and policies particularly during the last fifteen years, but indeed before them as well. Political attention, media commentary and social policy formulation has increasingly focused on the problems generated for society by specific groups of the population who are most likely to be poor or who abuse the welfare system.'

Evidence continues to mount on the widening gap between rich and poor, such as the report of the Inquiry into Income and Wealth published by the Joseph Rowntree Foundation in February 1995 which showed that the proportion of the population with less than half the average income trebled between 1977 and 1992. Nevertheless, the influence of this perception of the 'non-deserving poor' can be seen in the development of policies focusing particularly on individuals who are poor, rather than on the causes of poverty, and often involving proposals for further cuts and restrictions on welfare spending and stronger law and order measures to contain those who fail to conform to accepted values and behaviour. In 1993–94, the government mounted a stringent campaign to root out benefit fraud and abuse which the Social Security Secretary, Peter Lilley (1994), declared to be 'one of our top priorities'. The Incapacity for Work Bill, for example, removed eligibility for sickness and invalidity benefits for nearly 300,000 recipients who were then forced onto the unemployment register. In introducing the bill, Lilley declared that the bill was not an attack on sick and disabled people, but was designed to protect their benefit against those who abuse it and that anyone who is really concerned about the sick and disabled must be prepared to tackle the abuse of benefits which were meant for them. During the same year, other measures introduced to tackle benefit fraud and abuse included regulations to control 'benefit tourism' whereby claimants have to establish that they are habitually resident in this country before key benefits can be paid, a pilot scheme to enable the Department of Social Security and local authorities to exchange and cross-check information to reduce multiple claims and a three-year, £300 million programme to introduce benefit payment cards, more checks on new claims and increased reviews of existing claims. These were accompanied by increasingly firm declarations of intent to rethink social policy and the benefits system as a means of supporting the institution of the two-parent family rather than lone parenthood and calls by the Prime Minister for the law to be used more rigorously to keep beggars off the streets.

Defining need

So far, we have considered need as a relative concept in relation to poverty and have seen that poverty is itself a relative concept – relative, that is, to the norms of society. Thus, an individual's needs must be defined in relation to those of their peer group. In assessing need, it would be inappropriate to compare the needs of a person today with those of someone of the same age forty years ago, or indeed with those of someone living in another, perhaps poorer, society. Furthermore, as a relative concept, need is more than simply a matter of adequate nutrition or housing ('absolute' need). It embraces a much wider area of social life and is really about a person's ability to take part in all those aspects of life in which an average citizen of that society could reasonably expect to participate. Clearly, there may be conflict between 'expert' or professional definitions of need and the views and experiences of those who are in need and, as with the issue of poverty, conflicts in perspectives and definitions have implications for social policy.

The attitudes of policy makers, professionals and the general public towards concepts of poverty and need are inevitably influenced by their own personal values and often reflect judgements about the underlying causes of need. As we have seen, these, in turn, determine the types of social policy response we would advocate. Those who believe that unemployment is largely the fault of the 'workshy', for instance, would see the reduction in payments of unemployment benefit from a year to six months in 1993 as a means of restoring work incentives. Others who hold that unemployment has little to do with unemployed people themselves but, far more importantly, reflects the state of the economy would argue for higher levels of government investment in the economy in order to create more employment opportunities.

Thus, the ways in which needs are defined in our society have important implications for the types and levels of need that are identified and consequently for the nature of the social policies developed to address those needs. They also have implications for the way in which the providers of welfare services implement social policy. So, when need is defined very narrowly, such as in relation to a person's physical condition, the social policy response may also be very narrow. A person who has had a double lower-limb amputation, for example, may have their principal need defined by a health care professional as the maintenance of mobility, with the response being the provision of a wheelchair. A social worker might recommend meals-on-wheels or even residential care. When you have completed this session, however, you should be aware of potential discrepancies between the needs defined by professional carers and those defined by the people for whom they care. A disabled person may, for instance, identify their greatest need as being to have more social contact or to feel less ostracised, a need that has arisen not so much because of that person's condition, but because of societal attitudes that result in disabled people having poor access to public transport, buildings and employment opportunities or feeling shunned by other people. In this case, however appropriate the professional response may be to an individual client, the wider need will remain unmet until there is both a broader social policy response, such as the Disability (Civil Rights) Bill that was blocked in Parliament in May 1994, and more positive attitudes towards disabled people.

As a further example, consider the contradictions that are often inherent in social policy responses to the needs of black people. The assimilationist or 'colour blind' approach to universal provision in which race or cultural diversity is deemed to make no difference to black people's needs may, in fact, mean that they are simply expected to use existing services that are geared to the needs of white people and to make no special demands on them. Where a cultural pluralism approach is adopted and the needs of different ethnic groups are recognised, however, they are often perceived as being 'special needs' that make extra demands on services or are reduced to cultural stereotypes that can mask the needs of individuals. In exploring the needs of black women in the maternity services, for example, Phoenix (1990) observes that:

> 'Stereotypes of Asian women's "low" pain threshold can mean that their responses to pain in childbirth are greeted with irritation and not taken seriously (Brent Community Health Council 1981). Similarly, assumptions about Afro-Caribbean women "just popping them out like peas" can predispose medical staff to categorize women of Afro-Caribbean origin as physically more geared to childbearing than white women, and so requiring less support and sympathy. The belief that black women's behaviour can most readily be explained by reference to their supposed cultural origins can also obscure the similarities between black and white women. For example, women's right to have their infant's father with them was a hard-won advance in obstetric practice. In many hospitals, however, it has ossified into practice in such a way that it is no longer just an available right but is deemed to be essential ... If Asian women do not have their male partners with them in labour, this tends to be perceived as a further indication of the "repressive" culture under which Asian women are stereotyped to live (Brent Community Health Council 1981). On the other hand, white women who are not accompanied by their male partners during labour are likely to be considered as individually (rather than culturally) deviant. Conversely, women of Asian origin whose children's fathers are present during birth are likely to be presumed to have abandoned their "Asian culture", because heterogeneity within black groups is not recognized.'

As Phoenix points out, cultural practices are not simply divided along colour lines but are a result of a complex interrelationship of such factors as class, geographical locality and historical period. Black people, like white people, have a diversity of cultural practices and people of different racial origin but similar class backgrounds are likely to share certain beliefs and cultural practices. The introduction of the Patient's Charter by the Department of Health in 1991, with its National Charter Standard on respect for privacy, dignity and religious and cultural beliefs, marks a recognition of the importance of responding to individual needs rather than to stereotypes. It does require, however, that service providers look closely at their own practice in identifying how this aspect of social policy is to be implemented.

In practice, the 'special needs' approach is often translated into a demand that may come from service providers, rather than from consumers themselves, for separate or additional provision of services designed specifically for people from ethnic minority communities. In the early 1980s, for example, there was concern about the very poor take-up rate for meals-on-wheels and other services amongst the black pensioner population in London. A group of professionals in one borough accordingly got together to discuss the problem and decided that the reason for the low uptake was that black people had special needs in relation to their diet. Consequently, an 'ethnic' meals-on-wheels service was set up at considerable expense, providing a range of ethnic meals. The take-up of this service was still very low, however, resulting in considerable embarrassment to the local authority concerned. Subsequent research on behalf of the Greater London Council (Ackers 1985) involving discussions with black pensioners themselves, as consumers, showed that one of the reasons why they were not making use of existing provision was simply a lack of information; many people did not know that the service existed or did not know that they were eligible. Amongst those who *did* know of the service, there was concern about the quality and degree of choice offered by the menus, but this concern was shared equally by white pensioners.

The following activity asks you to reflect on your understanding of the role of professionals in defining need and how this may affect people's experience of welfare provision.

ACTIVITY 36   ALLOW 5 MINUTES

Re-read the brief account above of the research on the response of black pensioners to the ethnic meals-on-wheels service and note down any issues that you feel point to important messages about need and the relationship between professionals and consumers in defining need.

Commentary

In the case of the meals-on-wheels service, the process by which the needs of the black pensioner population were defined in this borough was clearly inappropriate, even though well-intentioned. The service providers failed to consult the potential recipients of the service and relied entirely on their own perceptions of those needs and their assumptions about the best way of meeting them. If the starting point had been to talk to people in order to find out why they were not using the existing service and to find out what their requirements were, an expensive mistake could have been averted. A further important message to emerge from this study was the need for comprehensive, accessible information about the range of services available if people are to be empowered and enabled to make real choices.

This example illustrates the way in which the relevance and appropriateness of welfare services is not simply dependent on the social policy that causes them to be provided in the first place, but also on the way in which individuals' own beliefs about social policy issues shape their professional response to their clients. A great deal of progress has been made in both policy and practice since, in the NHS Management Inquiry (Department of Health & Social Security, 1983), Roy Griffiths, a former chairman of Sainsbury's, first proposed the use of market research techniques as a valid means of measuring patient satisfaction and identifying patients' needs and expectations. Nevertheless, the concept of service users as passive recipients rather than active consumers of services has by no means disappeared. All too often, welfare provision is still determined by the values of service providers and the nature of the services they can offer, rather than by the needs of the people for whom they are being provided.

In the remainder of this session, we shall focus on the issue of need in relation to disabled people, exploring the conflict between what they themselves define as their needs and what others, and particularly professionals, perceive their needs to be. In doing so, we shall see how different ways of defining needs in relation to disability have important implications for social policy.

The social construction of disability

The importance of the process by which needs are defined can clearly be seen in the demand by the disabled people's movement, Rights not Charity, that disabled people should be seen as people first, rather than being defined by a medical condition such as multiple sclerosis, arthritis or cerebral palsy. Since the early 1980s, disabled people have become increasingly vocal and critical of the services offered to them, not only by local authorities and central government but also by voluntary agencies that have traditionally promoted their needs. Activists such as Finkelstein (1980) and Oliver (1983; 1990) have been influential in demonstrating how the needs of disabled people are often not met because they are defined in terms of the medical model which emphasises their medical needs, rather than the social model which focuses on their social needs.

To illustrate the distinction between the two models, consider the example of a person with cerebral palsy and the way in which their disablement may depend not only on the severity of their condition but also on the attitudes of society towards them. They may be unable to go to the local school or to join in local social activities without feeling humiliated or isolated. They may be unable to make use of the local swimming pool, not because of their impairment but because of the lack of wheelchair access and suitable changing facilities. Thus, they may not be disabled as much by their medical condition as by the attitudes of other people.

The theory underpinning the medical model borrows from bereavement counselling and views disability as a loss; as Oliver (1983) observes, it can be described as 'the personal tragedy theory of disability', a theory that is often at odds with disabled people's own perceptions of themselves and the world in which they live. The traditional emphasis on this model has perpetuated the image of disabled people as being reliant on professional help and incapable of an independent life. In contrast, the social model highlights the ways in which the attitudes and actions of society discriminate against disabled people and, in fact, actually disable people. It focuses attention on how society is organised by able-bodied people and the role of planners, architects, educators and health and social care professionals in creating an environment that largely excludes and restricts access by disabled people, effectively segregating them. It raises questions about issues such as physical access to buildings, the availability of suitable toilet facilities in shopping centres and workplaces, and about the attitudes of employers in their recruitment policies and of the general public towards increased social contact with disabled people. Why, for example, is there so often resistance to the siting of community homes for disabled people on residential housing estates? Perhaps most importantly, it challenges the way in which disabled people are largely excluded from decision-making about their own lives and from participation in the plannning of services that are supposedly designed to meet their needs.

By focusing on the social construction of disability, the social model seeks to support disabled people in articulating their own needs, identifying how they can best be met and asserting their autonomy and independence. In other words, it is concerned with empowerment. Lonsdale (1990) defines independence as 'being able to determine and take responsibility for one's life' and, in discussing the processes that can limit this independence and generate or encourage dependency, suggests that:

> 'In the presence of a physical disability this is more than likely to involve relying on help in the form of aids and appliances, housing and workplace adaptations, and personal assistance for day-to-day living. All these things, however, can be provided in different ways. Individuals can be coerced into dependency in return for financial and other forms of help. Or they can get help which deliberately promotes or increases autonomy and self-determination. Obstacles to independence can be both structural and ideological. Physical dependency, *per se*, need not impose a state of dependency on someone, but an unaccommodating and hostile environment will

certainly do so. Independence is not only a function of individual abilities, but the interaction between those abilities and the environment – physical and social.'

Thus, different forms of welfare intervention and, more specifically, different models of professional practice in relation to disabled people can have very different outcomes. Some forms of practice, particularly those paternalistic practices that operate on the premise of 'the professional knows best', promote dependency. In a research study on unmet need and the 1986 Disabled Person's Act (Ackers *et al.*, 1989), for example, the issue of risk-taking in relation to people with learning difficulties emerged frequently. A local work unit for disabled people was specifically designed and staffed to accommodate people with learning difficulties and provided an interesting and stimulating environment and, importantly, an escape from the home. Many parents and professionals were so cautious in their attitudes towards independence, however, that some families refused to permit their children to attend the unit or to travel alone on public transport. Another example concerned the attitudes of staff in a local residential home who were reluctant to allow the residents to attend meetings of a newly-established self-advocacy group in the local town, one of an increasing number of groups being set up and run by disabled people themselves, often with financial support from local authorities. Such over-cautious behaviour may actually deny disabled people their autonomy and foist on them a level of dependency, even though the carers may have the best possible intentions.

Our approach to the issue of disability, then, has clear implications for the nature and outcomes of social policy intervention. The dominance of the traditional medical model that deals with disability according to the medical categorisation of the specific impairment, is reflected in a dearth of literature in the social sciences on the process of disablement. Two exceptions to this are Lonsdale's *Women and Disability* (1990) and Oliver's *The Politics of Disablement* (1990), both of which specifically aim to shift the emphasis away from the medicalisation of disability and towards an understanding of society's role in influencing the experiences of disabled people.

In response to the weakness of the medical model, Wood (1981) devised a schema that outlines the relationship between disease, impairment, disability and handicap and highlights the role that society plays in the experience of disablement:

Disease: the underlying medical condition

Impairment: parts or systems of the body that do not work

Disability: things people cannot do, such as walking or dressing

Handicap: social and economic disadvantages.

This schema has subsequently developed into what is now known as the ICIDH (International Classification of Impairments, Disabilities and Handicaps) and has been adopted by the World Health Organization. According to this classification, impairment, disability and handicap become different stages in the disablement process and social policy intervention can take place at each stage with different results. For example, an individual may be impaired without being disabled – their inability to walk may be compensated by the provision of a suitable wheelchair – or may be disabled without being handicapped: visually impaired students, for example, can undertake courses if learning materials are produced in large print or Braille or on audio or video-tape. Such a model opens the way for analyses of the relationship between disablement and other social variables such as social class, gender, culture, family structure and sexuality. A black disabled woman, for example, may face triple discrimination in her efforts to gain employment because of her race, her gender and her disability. You may find it interesting to refer to the texts by Oliver (1990, Chapter 5), and Lonsdale (1990, Chapter 3) for a discussion of these relationships.

We can see from this schema that the extent to which an individual is disabled or handicapped is dependent not only on their disease or impairment but, perhaps more importantly, on variables such as prevailing social attitudes, their income, access to services and family support. The specific impact of an impairment may be related to the nature of a person's occupation (the ability to progress in their career, for example), or to the availability of voluntary sector support from organisations such as the Royal National Institute for the Blind, MIND or RADAR (the Royal Association for Disability and Rehabilitation). Depending upon these social factors, it is possible that an individual with only a mild impairment may be severely handicapped, whereas another person with a more severe impairment may experience considerably less handicap. For example, about half a million disabled people have wheelchairs and a government inquiry in 1986 concluded that dual-purpose wheelchairs for indoor and outdoor use should be made available, particularly to those without a companion. Nevertheless, although state funding is available in Scotland, wheelchair users in England, Wales and Northern Ireland must buy them themselves or obtain help from charities. As the executive director of the Muscular Dystrophy Group observed, 'the state might just as well issue an armchair as a manual wheelchair to a person with no upper-body strength' (Brindle, 1993b).

Since the ICIDH schema was developed, there has been a further shift in concepts of disability as disabled people themselves have seized the initative in defining their needs and identifying ways in which they should be met. In 1991, for example, the British Association of Social Workers unanimously passed a motion recognising disability as a form of social oppression rather than a state or condition. CCETSW, the Central Council for Education and Training in Social Work, issued guidance on disability issues in social work education and training which had been developed by a working group that was largely composed of representatives of organisations of disabled people (Stevens, 1991). The group specifically chose not to use the term 'handicap' since organisations of disabled people themselves reject it because of the implication of an additional burden or restriction. Instead, they agreed the following definitions of key words:

> **Disability**: the disadvantage or restriction of activity caused by contemporary social organisation which takes no or little account of people who have impairments and thus excludes them from activities.

> **Disabled person**: someone who as a consequence of their impairment experiences social oppression of whatever kind.

> 'Disability' informs a disabled person's perspective on society to the extent that it is a cultural perspective.

> **Disablism**: a form of social oppression or prejudice towards disabled people.

Thus, from a policy-making point of view, the greatest benefit of the social model is that it helps us to see that social policy can come into play at any or all of the stages between disease and handicap, with different implications for disabled people. Clearly, medical intervention at the initial 'disease' stage is important if the illness can be cured or its further development can be prevented. But this does not mean that medical intervention is always desirable.

ACTIVITY 37   ALLOW 10 MINUTES

Medical technology now exists that enables plastic surgery techniques to be used to conceal or reduce the physical manifestations of Down's syndrome. What arguments might be invoked here in favour of, and against, such intervention?

Commentary

You may feel that a child would benefit from advances in treatment that will enable him or her to look more 'normal' and therefore less vulnerable to stigmatisation. On the other hand, it may be important for people to recognise that a person with Down's syndrome has particular learning difficulties and that changing their appearance would not help them to overcome their other problems. You may also feel that such forms of intervention further promote a very narrow view of beauty or, at least, acceptable appearance which is essentially about conformity and does nothing to increase society's acceptance of people who look different.

There is clearly much still to be achieved in the prevention and treatment of chronic diseases such as arthritis and osteoporosis and one can only welcome advances such as immunisation that have virtually eliminated diseases such as rubella and poliomyelitis, especially in the Western world. In the majority of cases, however, such technical solutions are not possible. Wood (1981) therefore concludes that:

> ' ... provided the appropriate medical input is ensured, one can see
> that the major impact on residual disability will inevitably depend on
> societal response.'

It is clear from this discussion, therefore, that the needs of disabled people can be defined in different ways and with very different consequences. A professional needs assessment procedure that is based on the medical problem is likely to evoke a service-led – rather than a needs-led – response that may be very limited in scope ranging, for example, from the provision of aids and adaptations to day or residential care. As Meredith (1993) cautions:

> ' … people are often referred to in terms of "client groups". This is a kind of shorthand which focuses on the particular characteristics of groups of people. There is, however, a danger in thinking about people as belonging to client groups: in general, people do not think of themselves as carrying such a label … Lumping people into categories may adversely affect the kind of treatment or services they receive. A person aged over 65 could be physically disabled *and* have a mental illness. If he or she is mainly treated as being "elderly" mentally ill, they may not be thought of as eligible for services which are meant mainly for people who have physical disabilities. Services for people with mental health problems may include counselling, which may not be on offer to people who are labelled as *"elderly mentally ill"*.'

Health and social care workers committed to the social model would focus much more on working with clients to identify what they perceive their needs to be and how they, and their carers, can achieve their objectives. In a research study on the unmet needs of disabled people that was conducted for the social services department in Plymouth, for example, the most pressing needs expressed by the disabled people who were interviewed were for more social contact, better information on the availability of services and improved transport (Ackers *et al.*, 1989). Stevens (1991) emphasises that:

> 'It should not be assumed that needs are within the individual and the social work task is merely to identify them. A social work analysis could find that the needs arise from inaccessible environments or lack of resources. Self-assessment should be central to the assessment process and subsequent planning and evaluation should start from the same stand-point; in other words, disabled people are the best definers of their own needs.'

The adoption of a social model of disability thus shifts the emphasis of social policies from dealing with the effects of disability on an individual level to addressing the wider causes. In examining the link between impairment and disability, therefore, it is important to be fully aware of the impact of such factors as the structure of the built environment, the design of transport systems and employment practices, as well as the way in which resources are allocated. Ultimately, such an analysis raises important issues about the extent to which disabled people are able to participate actively in identifying needs and influencing policy at national and local level, both within the statutory sector and voluntary organisations. Only when this has been achieved can a real process of negotiation commence that involves disabled people – as people first and not as categories of impairment – in the definition of their own personal needs. The final activity asks you to consider the implications for future professional practice.

ACTIVITY 38　　　　　　　　　ALLOW **20** MINUTES

Read *Resource 10*, *'A last civil rights battle'* by Ryan (1988). Note down what is new about the concept of Centres for Integrated Living (CIL) and the reasons why they might be seen to challenge existing professional practice.

Commentary

The CIL concept is new in that it represents the collective interests of disabled people acting together to work for changes in the current pattern of service delivery. In particular, CILs demand more involvement in decision-making in relation to the planning and delivery of services. While they support the provision of welfare by the state, they do not wish to be passive recipients of care packages designed by able-bodied people on their behalf, but want to play an active role in the articulation of their own needs.

This approach could be seen as potentially threatening to health and social care professionals in that it questions their authority to make decisions about what people need and requires that they work more closely with their clients who are increasingly refusing to be passive recipients of services. As CCETSW (Stevens, 1991) acknowledges:

'Working with and for clients does not necessarily give them any control of their situation; it could just as easily perpetuate dependence. Social workers seeking to empower a user of services should therefore demonstrate that they can clarify the choices available to disabled people. Social workers are often gatekeepers to finite resources. Real empowerment, however, requires resource-based decisions to be shared with the individual. This does not mean that social workers should deny their responsibility for such decisions. Nor does it imply that social workers will be deskilled by this practice. While social workers should be able to facilitate the process of empowerment, their function is not to deliver empowerment as you would a bath aid. Empowerment means individuals or groups taking control of the decision-making processes, not doing things entirely for themselves. The aim is autonomy not independence: e.g. "I want to decide what socks I want to put on and when I want them put on but not necessarily to put them on myself." Empowerment implies the sharing of all information: e.g. about service and resources available, organizational structures, personal information and legal rights and entitlements and appeals procedures.'

Changing approaches to professional practice have been supported by developments in social policy that have resulted in considerable revisions to the way in which services are planned and delivered. Legislation such as the Disabled Persons (Services, Consultation and Representation Act) 1986, the Disabled Persons (Northern Ireland) Act 1989, the Children Act 1989 and the NHS and Community Care Act 1990 has been accompanied by policy initiatives such as the Patient's Charter which are all designed to ensure that services are more responsive to the needs of service users.

Nevertheless, disabled people are having to fight against wider policy changes that could undermine some of the progress that has been made and threaten to limit their growing independence. In 1994, for instance, new tax charges were imposed on essential adaptations made to company cars to enable them to be driven by disabled drivers, with employers being required to pay extra National Insurance contributions on the value of the car. This move was shortly followed by threats to the Priority Suppliers Scheme which gives Remploy, a major employer of disabled people, a second chance to bid for government contracts if other bids are lower. Clearly, both moves could seriously jeopardise employment opportunities for disabled people and force them into increased reliance on welfare services. At the same time, the economic welfare of low-income families of people with learning difficulties has come under threat with the decision of a growing number of local authorities to levy weekly fees, and meals and transport charges for their attendance at day centres, even though disability benefits are paid on the basis that such services are free. The day centres, which place particular emphasis on social learning, are gradually replacing adult training centres where, in the past, people with learning difficulties were generally paid a small wage for the work they did. Thus, the nature and extent of the services required by disabled people may be determined as much by wider social and economic policies as by their individual needs.

The civil rights battle has now been taken further than the level of local authority social services departments, health care provider units and voluntary organisations. In May 1994, the Minister for Disabled People was accused of filibustering tactics that effectively killed the Disability (Civil Rights) Bill in what was widely seen as being a reaction against the projected costs of its implementation. While the Bill failed on that occasion, despite the support of over 350 MPs, the fact that it had even been presented to Parliament is witness to the power of disabled people who had challenged the right of others to define their needs and, in the process had forced politicians, professionals and the general public to look beyond traditional models of care and support. In doing so, they succeeded in demonstrating not only the complex nature of disability, but also how a broad social policy response that goes far beyond the provision of services is required in order to meet the needs of disabled people and enable them to play a fuller role in the society in which they live. Their experience is a further illustration of the way in which different aspects of social policy interrelate at all levels to affect the experience of service users and shows how positive developments in one area may be hampered or compromised by policy changes in another.

In conclusion

Your work on this unit should have helped you to recognise the complexity of contemporary social policy and the way in which it shapes the lives of all members of our society. In particular, it should have underlined the importance of the interaction between different areas of government policy, including economic policy, and demonstrated why the study of social policy involves more than simply an awareness of services provided by government within the welfare state.

The unit should also have encouraged you to think about the importance of the wide range of welfare providers, from the family to the voluntary and private sectors. If we exclude consideration of these important areas of provision, we are left with only a partial view of the impact of social welfare on people's lives. In particular, by concentrating only on the statutory sector, we could be left with a very narrow view of the welfare state as being inherently benevolent and redistributive in favour of poorer sections of society. As you have seen, there has been a major shift away from statutory provision to the contracting of services from the private and voluntary sectors and a greater reliance on family carers. Looking at the various welfare sectors together, we can see how the redistributive effects of social policy are complex, often benefiting middle-income groups more than lower-income groups, and how, in practice, the role of social policy is not primarily about meeting need. As we have seen in this final session on the difficulties involved in identifying need, the definitions of need embedded within the perspectives of policy makers or the practice of welfare professionals often tend to create or foster dependency rather than to empower service users.

It is with this important issue in mind that you should now be better able to analyse critically your future role as a health or social care professional within the mixed economy of welfare and to recognise both how your own professional practice is influenced by broader social policy and the way in which this impinges on the lives of the people you are there to support.

Summary

1 Need is a relative concept that must be defined in relation to the prevailing norms of society and that embraces all those aspects of life in which citizens of that society could reasonably expect to participate.

2 The way in which concepts of need are defined in our society has important implications for the kinds and levels of need identified and consequently for the nature of social policy responses.

3 The social model of disability shifts the emphasis of social policy from interventions to deal with the effects of disability on an individual level to addressing the wider causes.

Before you move on, check that you have achieved the objectives given at the beginning of this session and, if not, review the appropriate sections.

LEARNING REVIEW

Before you started work on this unit, you were asked to complete a learning profile to assess your current level of knowledge and identify key areas on which you particularly needed to focus. Now that you have completed the unit, use the list of anticipated learning outcomes to review the progress you have made during your study of contemporary social policy. These are repeated below.

For each outcome, tick the box that most closely corresponds to the point you feel you have now reached and compare it with your responses in the learning profile. If there are any areas that you still find difficult to understand, you should find it helpful to review the sessions concerned and to discuss any remaining problems with your tutor.

	Not at all	Partly	Quite well	Very well

Session One

I can:

- define social policy ☐ ☐ ☐ ☐
- outline three main perspectives on the functions of social policy ☐ ☐ ☐ ☐
- identify the key sectors involved in welfare provision ☐ ☐ ☐ ☐
- distinguish between the ways in which different socio-economic groups benefit most from the welfare state. ☐ ☐ ☐ ☐

Session Two

I can:

- identify factors contributing to overall improvements in health in the UK ☐ ☐ ☐ ☐
- summarise the evidence for the persistence of inequalities in health ☐ ☐ ☐ ☐
- outline the major explanations for inequalities in health ☐ ☐ ☐ ☐
- discuss the potential contribution of the Health of the Nation initiative to a reduction in inequalities in health. ☐ ☐ ☐ ☐

Session Three

I can:

- describe the roles of the four main sectors in the mixed economy of welfare ☐ ☐ ☐ ☐

	Not at all	Partly	Quite well	Very well

Session Three *continued*

- outline the provisions of the NHS and Community Care Act 1990

| | ☐ | ☐ | ☐ | ☐ |

- identify the providers of community care services in my local area.

| | ☐ | ☐ | ☐ | ☐ |

Session Four

I can:

- identify examples of social policy that reflect specific political ideologies

| | ☐ | ☐ | ☐ | ☐ |

- outline Conservative Party ideology on the role of the statutory sector

| | ☐ | ☐ | ☐ | ☐ |

- outline Labour Party ideology on the role of the statutory sector

| | ☐ | ☐ | ☐ | ☐ |

- discuss the advantages and disadvantages of universal and selective welfare provision.

| | ☐ | ☐ | ☐ | ☐ |

Session Five

I can:

- assess the impact of the shift towards private sector provision on the role of the state

| | ☐ | ☐ | ☐ | ☐ |

- identify the advantages and disadvantages of the emphasis on home-ownership in contemporary housing policy

| | ☐ | ☐ | ☐ | ☐ |

- discuss the implications of the growth in private health care and the introduction of the internal market to the NHS for consumer choice, the quality of services and equality of access.

| | ☐ | ☐ | ☐ | ☐ |

Session Six

I can:

- describe the range and scope of voluntary sector involvement in the provision of welfare

| | ☐ | ☐ | ☐ | ☐ |

- review some ideas and ideologies underpinning the expansion of the voluntary sector, in particular the notion of altruism or giving freely to others

| | ☐ | ☐ | ☐ | ☐ |

	Not at all	Partly	Quite well	Very well

Session Six *continued*

- assess the role of voluntarism and its place within social policy ☐ ☐ ☐ ☐
- suggest areas where voluntary sector involvement may be most appropriate. ☐ ☐ ☐ ☐

Session Seven

I can:

- identify the main categories of task undertaken by carers ☐ ☐ ☐ ☐
- discuss the advantages and disadvantages of informal and institutional care ☐ ☐ ☐ ☐
- discuss the significance of the gender of carers in determining the level of support provided ☐ ☐ ☐ ☐
- recognise potential constraints on the expansion of the informal sector. ☐ ☐ ☐ ☐

Session Eight

I can:

- discuss need as a relative concept ☐ ☐ ☐ ☐
- suggest why the way in which needs are defined has important implications for social policy ☐ ☐ ☐ ☐
- discuss how the definitions of need adopted by health and social care professionals can affect the experiences of those for whom they care. ☐ ☐ ☐ ☐

RESOURCES SECTION

Contents

RESOURCE I

Equal Opportunities Policy, University of Plymouth, 1993

University of Plymouth Equal Opportunities Policy Statement

"The University of Plymouth will provide a working and learning environment that is free of discrimination and encourages equality of opportunity"

Equal Opportunities Policy

1. Introduction

The University of Plymouth is an Equal Opportunities employer and is committed to the promotion of Equal Opportunities for all its staff, students and applicants. It affirms its intention to pursue policies and practices which do not discriminate against any groups or individuals, either directly or indirectly, on the grounds of gender, race, colour, disability, religion, age, occupation, marital status, or sexual orientation.

The Deputy Vice-Chancellor (Secretarial) has responsibility for ensuring compliance with relevant legislation and promotion of good practice in Equal Opportunities matters.

Staff and students of the University of Plymouth are required to comply with this policy and with relevant legal requirements, and are expected to promote a culture of equality of opportunity. Any incidents of discrimination or harassment will be investigated and may be grounds for expulsion or dismissal. Appropriate training and development will be provided to assist staff in implementing this policy and promoting an appropriate culture.

2. Definitions

2.1 Direct Discrimination occurs when a person of one category (for example a female) is treated less favourably on the grounds of that category, than a person of another category (for example males) would be treated in the same (or not materially different) circumstances.

2.2 Indirect Discrimination occurs when a requirement or condition is applied equally to categories, but

2.2.1 The proportion of one category (for example females) is considerably smaller than the proportion of another category (for example males) which can comply, and

2.2.2 which cannot be shown to be justifiable irrespective of the category of the person concerned, and

2.2.3 which is to the person's detriment. For example: a recruitment advertisement requiring applicants to be six feet tall.

3. Students

3.1 Access – all appropriately qualified students and potential students will be given equal consideration for selection for courses, having regard to the nature of the University's buildings and other environmental limitations.

3.2 Selection – entry qualifications for courses will only include those that are necessary and justifiable. All selection processes will be thorough, carried out objectively, and will only address the applicant's suitability for the course and ability to fulfil the course requirements. Staff involved in selection processes will be trained to achieve these ends.

3.3 Curricula – it will be the responsibility of Deans, Heads, Course Leaders, and all other members of staff who set and teach curricula and syllabi, to avoid bias in these areas. Learning materials should be non-discriminatory; if discriminatory material is used to make a point, the discriminatory nature should be pointed out by the staff member using the material.

3.4 Learning Conditions – the University will take account of the needs of individual students and, wherever reasonably practicable within existing constraints, consideration will be given to issues, such as catering for dependants, when lectures and examinations are timetabled.

3.5 Advice – counselling and advice for students, on issues such as discrimination and harassment, will be available from the Student Services Centre.

4. Staff

4.1 Access – all staff and applicants for jobs will be given equal consideration for selection, promotion and training as appropriate, taking person specifications into account. A Recruitment Monitoring Form will be sent with all application forms, but will be used only for monitoring purposes and not in the selection process.

4.2 Selection and promotion – shortlisting and interviewing processes will be thorough, carried out objectively and will avoid bias (staff involved in these processes will be trained to achieve these ends). Interview panels will wherever reasonably practicable include both genders. Shortlisting/Interviewing Monitoring Forms will be used in the selection process.

4.3 Working conditions – the University will take account of the needs of the individual members of staff and, wherever reasonably practicable, will use flexitime and/or special contractual terms to assist with issues such as disabilities, religious observance and caring for dependants.

4.4 Staff Development – the University will not discriminate on the grounds mentioned in paragraph 1, in the provision of training and development to assist staff to perform their jobs effectively and to achieve their own personal development. Training and development of individual members of staff will be recorded and monitored.

4.5 Advice – counselling and advice for staff, on the law relating to Equal Opportunities and on the issues of discrimination and harassment, will be available from the Personnel Department.

5. Advertising and Information

5.1 All University advertisements and publications will demonstrate its commitment to Equal Opportunities. Zlanguage and positive images, and will give clear requirements for entry to courses and details of facilities available.

5.2 Information regarding new and promoted posts will be circulated throughout the institution. Posts will be advertised externally unless there are justifiable reasons to do otherwise.

6. Facilities

The University will, wherever reasonably practicable, provide facilities, such as specialised equipment and food, to allow equal access by all staff, students and applicants to the education and employment it provides.

7. Monitoring and Review

The Deputy Vice-Chancellor (Secretarial) will oversee the monitoring of this policy to ensure its effectiveness and, together with the Equal Opportunities network, will review the policy annually. Action by Deans and Heads to implement the Policy will be reviewed as part of the appraisal process.

8. Publication

This policy will be published by the Vice-Chancellor and drawn to the attention of all staff, students and other interested parties. Copies will be issued to current and new staff and students, and will be available from the Personnel Department, the Student Services Centre and the Student's Union.

9. Responsibility

The Deputy Vice-Chancellor (Secretarial) is responsible for implementing this policy. Advice and information on Equal Opportunities implementation and problems can be sought from him/her, the personnel Department, the Student Services Centre or Equal Opportunities Network members (a list of current members can be obtained form the Personnel Department).

Why do we need such a policy at all?

Every organisation needs to make the best use of the skills and abilities of all members of its staff. This is good management as it helps an organisation and its staff to get the greatest benefit from their education and training. It also serves to improve motivation and performance which helps to reduce staff turnover.

In the UK today almost half of the workforce is female; our society is multi-racial and people with disabilities who can, and want to, make a full contribution in the workplace, are also a part of that society.

The number of 18 year olds in the population will have fallen from 900,000 to 600,000 in the period 1981 to 1995, resulting in a shrinking recruitment market place. Employers who discriminate against certain groups of staff will reduce this market place even further and are also unlikely to retain their best employees.

The University of Plymouth wants to be a good employer. It wants to ensure that people from all groups in our society are given the opportunity to contribute to its success and that they are not prevented from doing so by artificial and unnecessary barriers.

Discrimination is also unlawful. Employers and employees who practice discrimination may find themselves involved in litigation.

What are the likely benefits to me?

The main benefit is that there will be greater fairness in the way that job applicants are treated. People will be considered on the basis of their ability to do a job or cope with increased responsibilities; this will benefit everyone in the University in due course.

What are the main components of the policy?

The policy will primarily address issues concerned with gender, ethnic minorities and people with disabilities.

What are the issues concerned with gender?

The University employs a large number of women most of whom work in administrative and manual jobs. Some of our teaching departments have a surprisingly low number of women lecturers; they are attempting to recruit women students but do not have the staff who can act as successful role models. With a few notable exceptions, women are not widely represented in the senior academic posts – there are historical reasons for this but, it does lead to a perception, be it correct or not, that our University is a male dominated institution.

What are the issues concerned with ethnic minorities?

Our students will live and work in a society which is multi-racial and multi-cultural. In the UK as a whole, ethnic minorities comprise some 6% of the population. Locally, this figure is around 0.9% of the population whilst approximately 0.5% of our staff are drawn from these groups. As a University we should be leading the field locally in creating a working and learning environment which reflects the ethnic and cultural diversity which is a fact of life in British society.

What are the issues concerned with people with disabilities?

The law requires every employer to employ a number of people with disabilities; at present this figure is 3% of the total number of staff. Less than 1% of our staff are registered disabled and we have to apply every six months for an Exemption Certificate from the Department of Employment. Many people with disabilities could make full contribution to the working life of the University and we need to ensure that they do not suffer from unfair discrimination when they apply for jobs.

RESOURCE 2

Woolley and Le Grand, 'The Ackroyds, the Osbornes and the welfare state: the impact of the welfare state on two hypothetical families over their life-times', Policy and Politics, 1990

The Ackroyds, The Osbornes and the Welfare State:
the impact of the welfare state on two hypothetical families over their life-times

This paper is a study of fiscal incidence, but a rather unusual one. Instead of attempting to determine the impact of the welfare state on a representative sample survey, it attempts to assess that impact on two hypothetical families over their life-times: the working class Ackroyds and the middle class Osbornes. It examines the amounts the families receive in cash benefits, the costs of the social services they use and the value of the taxes they pay to finance those benefits. It concludes that, while cash benefits except old age pensions benefit the Ackroyds more than the Osbornes, pensions and social services overwhelmingly favour the Osbornes. However, when finance is taken into account, the system as a whole may redistribute income.

Introduction

In this paper we describe the impact of the welfare state on two hypothetical families over their life-times: the working class Ackroyds and the middle class Osbornes. The work was undertaken in an attempt to put some flesh on the bones of fiscal incidence studies that are generally heavily statistical – to give some feel for what the numbers derived from such studies might actually mean to individual families. As such, the methodology is unconventional for a piece of social science research; in particular, we can obviously make no claim for the representativeness of the 'sample'. We believe, nonetheless, that the results shed light on the general question of the redistributive impact of the welfare state, and do so in a more novel, and perhaps more entertaining, fashion than many more conventional studies.

In what follows, we examine for the Ackroyds and Osbornes:

–the amounts the families receive through various cash benefits (old age pension, invalidity pension, housing benefit, sickness benefit and statutory sick pay, supplementary benefit and unemployment benefit)

–the benefits they get from welfare-related tax reliefs (mortgage interest, private pensions, private education)

–the use they make of various social services (the National Health Service, the education system, housing, public transport and the subsidised performing arts)

–the taxes they pay to finance these benefits and services.

In the rest of the paper, we present first the life histories of the two families. We then discuss the extent to which they are typical and offer some comments on the paper's approach. The final section summarises the results. An Appendix provides details of their construction.

Life Histories

Here we present the life histories of the two families. They are, we believe, not unrealistic representatives of their respective classes. The histories, however, are unrealistic in one key respect: the social and economic context in which they begin (that corresponding to the mid-1980s) is assumed to remain unchanged for the remainder of the relevant individuals' lives. The justification for this assumption is discussed below.

The Ackroyds

We first meet Jim Ackroyd on his wedding day. Jim, aged 23, is marrying Tracy, aged 21, with whom he has been going out for four years. Both were born and bred in Salford. Jim is a fork-lift operator in a light engineering factory. After the wedding, Jim and Tracy move in with Tracy's parents but have their name down on the council's housing list for a flat. Jim commutes to work by bus. A year later they have their first child, and eighteen months after that their second child is born.

After two and a half years of waiting, Jim and Tracy get a council flat. Jim continues to work at the engineering factory and still travels to work four miles each way by bus. By now he is earning the average wage for a fork-lift operator in the warehouse (around £150 per week in 1985/86). Although this is not enormous, it is high enough to render them ineligible for Family Income Supplement or housing benefit. They have few luxuries but watch a lot of television. Jim smokes around 20 cigarettes a day.

Jim and Tracy's children attend a local nursery school, then primary school, followed by a comprehensive secondary school. Both children leave school at sixteen, with two passes in GCSEs, and put in about six months on the Youth Training Scheme before looking for work.

The Ackroyds' financial situation improves when the children are in secondary school, and Tracy (now aged 35) takes a part time job as a sales clerk, earning £43 per week.

When Jim is 45 years old, he is made redundant when the firm he works for has to cope with a recession. He receives unemployment benefit for a year. The children, now 18 and 20, still live at home, and help out a little, and Tracy's wages contribute to the family income. However, when Jim's unemployment benefit runs out, Jim and Tracy apply for supplementary benefit to make ends meet.

After a year on supplementary benefit (two year's unemployment), Jim gets a job as a security guard for another local firm. The job is slightly better paid than the one he left, and Jim now earns £155 a week.

For some years Jim's chest has been giving him trouble, with smoking, manual work and damp housing taking their toll. When necessary, he goes to the doctor to get a medical certificate, but Jim is not very good at describing his symptoms, and the doctor does not realise the severity of Jim's problem. At the age of 56 he collapses at work and is taken to hospital, where he remains for four weeks. Emphysema is diagnosed and Jim has to give up work.

Now that Jim is unable to work, he is eligible for an invalidity pension. The pension and Tracy's earnings are their only sources of income. They now get housing benefit to help with the rent. After Tracy retires, the Ackroyds get by on Jim's retirement pension, supplemented by housing benefit.

Jim dies at age 68. Tracy outlives him by almost eight years, dying a few months after her seventy-fourth birthday.

The Osbornes

Stephen Osborne works in the City branch of a large firm of accountants. We first meet him when, at the age of 23, he has just passed his accountancy exams. Two years later he marries Henrietta, a teacher who is two years younger and is the daughter of one of the partners in his father's firm of solicitors. Henrietta and Stephen buy a small, picturesque house in a village in the Chilterns. Stephen commutes into London from High Wycombe railway station, while Henrietta teaches in the local state primary school.

When Henrietta is 26 she stops work to have their first child. Two years later they have their second. Both children start their education at the state nursery school, and then move on to the local primary school where Henrietta used to teach. At age 10 they enroll as day pupils in a private school nearby. At age 11 they take entrance exams, and are accepted into private boarding school. Henrietta now has time on her hands, and goes back to teaching part-time.

Stephen and Henrietta's favourite forms of entertainment are the theatre and the opera. They attend several performances a year, at the Royal Opera House in Covent Garden, the South Bank Centre or the Barbican.

Because of hard work and stress, Stephen has a heart attack at the age of 47, followed by another one the following year. After each heart attack he takes eight weeks off work. A heart by-pass operation is recommended, which is done on the National Health Service. After the operation, Stephen takes an extended vacation to recover, remaining off work for four months.

Stephen takes early retirement at age 62. He dies at age 73. He is outlived by Henrietta, who passes away shortly before her eightieth birthday.

Are these typical life histories?

The life histories are, in one sense, completely typical and, in another sense, quite unusual. The families are typical in that their life expectancy, number of children, education patterns, accommodation, recreation choices and so on are average for families in their socio-economic group. However, it is unusual for a family to be 'typical' in as many respects as the Ackroyds and the Osbornes are. For example, most people marry in their early twenties and do not get divorced, most people have two children, most men work for most of their lives and die around age 71, while most women work for some of their lives and die around age 77, with some variation according to socio-economic status. However, relatively few families conform exactly to this typical pattern – some couples get divorced, others have more or less than two children, some people die young and others live to a grand old age. The Ackroyds and the Osbornes are unusual in being so typical.

General approach

Why look at just two families?

The Ackroyds and the Osbornes are 'unusual' in being typical working and middle class families. It is not possible to use the Ackroyds and the Osbornes to assess the impact of the welfare state on all types of families, such as single parent families. Assessments of the overall impact of the welfare state have been produced by several authors, summarised in Le Grand (1982), and Goodin and Le Grand (1987). We will refer to this work throughout this paper.

The Central Statistical Office (CSO) pro-

duces biannual estimates of the impact of the welfare state on an 'average' family. However, unlike our calculations, they do not describe the benefits actually experienced by any family. For example, according to CSO (1986b), a low income family receives £217 child benefit annually. However, a simple calculation shows that, if a family receives child benefit for an entire year, the amount of benefit received is £364 per child. Very few families receive an odd amount of benefit such as £217.

A. B. Atkinson gives the following argument in favour of considering hypothetical families like the Ackroyds and the Osbornes: 'Hypothetical examples provide a convenient way of presenting the implications of changes in taxes and benefits. The man in the street can readily understand statements like 'the average worker will pay £x in extra taxes but receive £y in benefits' or that 'the scheme will pay £z a month extra to single parent families'. Such examples may be particularly helpful where the effects of the proposals are complex ...' (Atkinson, 1985 p.152).

Do the details of life history matter?

Differences in the details of life history may alter the timing of benefits over the life-cycle, the type and, in certain instances, the amount of benefits received. Consider, for example, two men, one of whom is unemployed for a year at age 20 and one who loses his job at age 30. The first will receive basic unemployment benefit and, if he is living on his own, may also receive housing benefit. The second, if he is married with children, will receive a greater amount of unemployment benefit, and may also receive housing benefit and supplementary benefit. The 30 year old receives different benefits, receives the benefits at a later stage in his life-cycle, and receives a greater amount of benefits than the 20 year old.

The unpredictable details of life history make little difference to the total amount of benefits received over the life-cycle. Far more significant are the predictably lower amounts of, for example, higher education benefits a working class family receives due to the low probability of a working class individual attending university, or the greater amount of pension received by a middle class family, because of the middle class's greater life expectancy. The most important determinants of the amount of benefits received over the life-cycle are the amount of time an individual spends in the labour force, his or her earnings capacity, and his or her tastes, particularly for education, travel and the arts.

Frozen in time?

The Ackroyds and the Osbornes live their

whole lives under the 1985/86 taxation and benefit regimes and, more generally, under the economic and social system prevailing at that time. This can be justified in two ways. First, one might think of the stories of the Ackroyds and the Osbornes as being prospective life histories: that is, the histories of the individuals in these families as if they were born today. Two questions then arise: why not take into account possible economic, demographic and social changes; and why not discount future benefits? To ask the first question is almost to answer it; it would be an enormous and probably fruitless task to attempt accurately to predict the course of all the possible factors that are likely to affect the lives of our two families over the next 70 years. The only reasonable thing to do, therefore, is to assume no change. The question of discounting seems irrelevant. As Rawls (1973, p.293) argues, 'The mere difference of location in time, of something's being earlier or later, is not in itself a rational ground for having more or less regard for it.' The only reason for discounting future benefits in this context would be that they are uncertain; but here we are assuming a certain future.

The second justification involves interpreting the Ackroyds' and Osbornes' life histories as a series of case studies. The Ackroyds and the Osbornes do not exist. Instead, they represent dozens of families, each at a different life stage, but with the same background and environment.

What do we mean by benefits?

Benefits are taken to include both direct expenditures and tax reliefs. There are two reasons for including tax reliefs in the welfare state. First, individuals do benefit as a result of tax reliefs. Second, tax reliefs can be viewed as equivalent to direct government expenditures, since they have exactly the same impact on the government's net fiscal position.

Benefits from particular programmes are valued at cost. They are assumed to be incident upon, and only upon, their nominal recipients. The analysis is partial, not general: in particular, individual behaviour is assumed to be independent of benefits received or of taxes paid. None of these is an innocuous assumption (see Le Grand, 1982 Appendix, and Goodin and Le Grand, 1987, Ch.2, for more extended discussions of the issues involved), but they are probably inevitable if any estimates are to be produced at all.

The unit of analysis is at the household level, beginning when Jim Ackroyd and Stephen Osborne are twenty-three. For Jim and Tracy, this coincides with their marriage. For Stephen and Henrietta, this coincides with Stephen passing his accountancy

exams. The household approach is equivalent to calculating the benefits experienced by the older generation over the whole life-cycle, if the life pattern of the younger generation follows that of the older generation.

Benefits are calculated with the system of taxes and benefits held at 1985/86 levels throughout. The year 1985/86 is the last for which all relevant data are available. The possible effect of changes in the State Earnings Related Pension Scheme (SERPS) is discussed in a concluding comment. Tax reliefs are calculated at the then basic rate of 27% throughout.

Results

The programmes investigated are;
Cash benefits, excluding retirement pensions
> Child benefit
> Family income supplement (FIS)
> Housing benefit
> Invalidity pension
> Sickness benefit
> Statutory sick pay
> Supplementary benefit
> Unemployment benefit

Retirement pensions
> Direct expenditures
> Tax reliefs for private pensions

Social Services
> National Health Service (NHS)
> Education: direct expenditures
> tax reliefs for private education
> Housing: mortgage interest tax relief
> Subsidies to public transport
> Subsidies to the arts

It should be noted that these by no means exhaust all forms of direct public expenditure, nor all tax reliefs. In particular, data limitations forced us to omit the following welfare and welfare-related programmes: personal social services, expenditure on highways, tax subsidies to company cars, libraries, the exemption of owner-occupied housing from capital gains tax and the age allowance.

Cash benefits excluding retirement pensions

Cash benefits, excluding retirement pensions, benefit the Ackroyds more than the Osbornes, as shown in Table 1. Most of the differences in benefits can be explained by the fact that Jim Ackroyd spends eleven of his possible working years either sick or unemployed, while Stephen Osborne is never unemployed, and spends a total of eight months off work due to illness.

The Ackroyds are not atypical in the amount of benefits they receive. The benefits are received for the most part, during the

11 years Jim is out of the labour force. It is quite usual to be sick or unemployed for eleven years – an average man is employed for just over 38 of the 49 years between school leaving and retirement age. By age 60, only 505 of men are working (calculated from OPCS, 1986, Table 6.2). Jim is unusual, however, in that he receives most of his benefits in the form of invalidity pension; more individuals receive unemployment benefit than invalidity pension (1.02m versus 0.8m).

The low level of benefits received by the Osbornes can be explained by Stephen's relatively good health and excellent employment record. Two points are worth noting here, however. First, the Osbornes receive more child benefit than the Ackroyds because their children are in school longer. Child benefit is received for children between sixteen and eighteen in full time education. Stephen Osborne receives more statutory sick pay both because sick pay is earnings related and because he receives it on three occasions, his two heart attacks and a heart bypass operation, while Jim receives it just once.

It should be noted that the numbers in Table 1 are calculated assuming 100% take-up rates. In other words, the Ackroyds and the Osbornes claim all the benefits to which they are entitled. If we assumed less than 100% take up for the means-tested benefits, the benefits received by the Ackroyds would be lower than those shown in Table 1. Estimated take up rates for most means-tested benefits are in fact considerably less than 100% (Atkinson, 1985, pp.78-82); so the results are likely to overestimate the Ackroyds' benefits.

Retirement pensions

The single largest welfare state expenditure is retirement pensions. Table 2 shows various estimates of the pension benefits received by the Ackroyds and the Osbornes. In all three estimates, Jim Ackroyd is covered by the national insurance retirement pension. In the first estimate, Stephen Osborne contracts into SERPS (State Earnings Relation Pension Scheme), while in the second two, Stephen contracts out. In the third estimate, Henrietta Osborne has her own retirement pension.

An inspection of Table 2 shows that the Osbornes receive substantially more retirement pension than the Ackroyds, regardless of whether or not Stephen contracts out of SERPS. The Osbornes simply live longer to take advantage of the benefits.

Social services

Welfare state programmes apart from cash benefits, such as education, health, transport subsidies, and subsidies to the arts, overwhelmingly favour the middle classes, as is shown in Table 3.

The estimates in Table 3 are conservative. The housing subsidy is estimated by taking basic rate relief on a mortgage which is average for the Osbornes' income group. The health estimates are based on equal expenditures for the Ackroyds and the Osbornes. The education estimates reflect the £5,500 per year expenditures the Osborne children receive during three years of university education.

The health care expenditures do not take into account the differential costs of the treatment received by Stephen Osborne, as

TABLE 1

Directly calculated cash benefits
(excluding retirement pensions)

	The Ackroyds	The Osbornes	Ratio of Ackroyds to Osbornes
	1985/86 benefit scales		
Child benefit	11,648	13,104	1.13
F.I.S.	nil	nil	-
Housing benefit	17,594	nil	-
Invalidity pension	28,222	nil	-
Sickness benefit	583	262	0.45
Statutory sick pay	240	1,064	4.43
Supplementary benefit	1,510	nil	-
Unemployment benefit	1,583	nil	-
Total	61,380	14,430	0.24

Source: Calculated using November 1985 benefit rates, given in DHSS (1986)

TABLE 2
Retirement pensions received

	Ackroyds	Osbornes
Estimate 1a	29,111	64,677
Estimate 2		
direct expenditures	29,111	43,613
tax reliefs		10,810b
		20,140c
Estimate 3		
direct expenditures	29,111	69,120
tax reliefs		10,810b
		20,140c

a For description of assumptions implicit in each estimate, see text.
b Not adjusted for size of contributions
c Adjusted for size of contributions (see Appendix)

there are no data available on the cost of given operations within the NHS. However, American research (Oster, Colditz and Kelly, 1984) estimates the cost of a heart bypass operation at $20,000 (1980, US$), and the cost of hospitalisation and follow-up after the first attack at $3,092 (1983 US$). In contrast, the cost of hospitalisation during an emphysema attack was estimated at $2,708 (1983, US$). The health expenditure figures also do not take into account differences in the quality of any treatment received by the Ackroyds and the Osbornes, or the frequency with which each is referred to outside specialists, both of which are likely to be higher for the latter. (Le Grand, 1982, pp. 26-30). Accordingly, it can be argued that they are a conservative estimate of the differences between the expenditures on the Ackroyds and the expenditures on the Osbornes.

The transport subsidy incorporates the 4.65 pence per mile subsidy Stephen Osborne receives during daily journeys to and from High Wycombe to London. Although the transport figure is surprising, it is not incompatible with other estimates, such as those in Le Grand (1982). If we make the not unreasonable assumption that the distribution of public subsidies follows the distribution of private expenditures, families in the top 10% of the income distribution receive ten times the rail subsidy that families in the bottom 10% receive.

The subsidy to the arts is another figure that is at first sight surprising but is ultimately plausible. The Osbornes are assumed to have an average entertainment budget for their income group, which they spend on the theatre, rather than sporting events or the cinema. They attend the theatre and the Royal Opera House at Covent Garden. Neither of these entertainments are as heavily subsidised as, for example, touring opera.

Total benefits

Table 4 shows all welfare state expendi-

TABLE 3
Social services benefits (1985/86)

	Ackroyds	Osbornes	Ratio of Ackroyds to Osbornes
Housing	nil	25,763	-
Health	38,180	43,766	1.15
Education			
Direct expenditure	24,210	43,676	1.80
Tax reliefs	nil	3,470	nil
Public transport	1,580	21,109	13.4
Arts subsidies	nil	8,758	-
Total	63,970	146,542	2.29

Sources: see Appendix

tures taken together. The pattern revealed is relatively simple, Cash benefits except pensions favour the Ackroyds. Direct expenditures (that is, excluding the value of tax reliefs) on pensions, health and education favour the Osbornes. Cash benefits and those direct expenditures together almost exactly cancel each other out. The Osbornes receive somewhat less benefits than the Ackroyds if Stephen contracts out of SERPS and Henrietta opts out of national insurance, but somewhat more benefits if Stephen remains in SERPS. This means that, if the welfare state was narrowly defined in terms of cash benefits and direct expenditures on health and education, its total life-time impact is broadly equal, with total benefits received of around £150,000.

If the welfare state is more correctly but still narrowly interpreted as including tax reliefs on pensions, education and housing, the Osbornes receive over £30,000 more welfare state benefits than the Ackroyds. If Stephen Osborne does not contract out of SERPS, the Osbornes receive £40,000 or 30% more welfare state benefits over their life-time than do the Ackroyds.

If the interpretation of the welfare state is extended to include the welfare-related activities of public transport and subsidies to the arts, the total impact becomes even more favourable to the Osbornes. The total lifetime benefits received by the Ackroyds in this broadly defined welfare state are £154,461, while those received by the Osbornes are between £215,395 and £225,649. The ratio of benefits received by the Osbornes to those received by the Ackroyds is, therefore, between 1.39 to 1.46

Does the welfare state redistribute income?

The answer to this question will depend on how the burden of finance of the welfare state is distributed: that is, who would received a tax reduction, and of what size, if all welfare programmes were abolished. This is not easy to estimate, since welfare programmes are, on the whole, not financed out of earmarked taxes but out of general tax revenues that also finance other, non-welfare, public expenditures. In these circumstances, to predict how people's tax burdens would change if the welfare state were abolished is at best a hit-and-miss affair (see Goodin and Le Grand, 1987, Chapter 2, for a detailed discussion).

One crude assumption is that every household's tax burden would be reduced by the same proportion as abolishing welfare programmes would reduce overall government expenditure (again, see Goodin and Le Grand, 1987, for an explanation of precisely how crude this assumption is). The Ackroyds pay £54,135 in income tax and national insurance contributions (19% of

TABLE 4
Summary of total benefits

	Ackroyds	Osborne's pension		Ratio of Ackroyds to Osbornes
		Estimate 1	Estimate 2	
	£	£	£	
Direct expenditures				
Cash benefits	61,380	14,430	14,430	0.24
Retirement pension	29,111	64,677	43,613	1.22/1.50
Health	38,180	43,766	43,766	1.15
Education	24,210	43,676	43,676	1.80
Total direct expenditure	152,881	166,549	145,485	1.09/0.95
Tax reliefs				
Housing	nil	25,763	25,763	
Retirement pension	nil	nil	10,810	
Education	nil	3,470	3,470	
Total tax reliefs	nil	29,233	40,043	
Total narrow welfare state	152,881	195,782	185,528	1.28/1.21
Public transport	1,580	21,109	21,109	13.4
Art subsidies	nil	8,758	8,758	
Total broad welfare state	154,461	225,649	215,395	1.46/1.39

life-time earnings) and £83,904 in other taxes (29% of life-time earnings). In 1985/86, 69.2% of government expenditures was allocated to the welfare state as defined in this paper. The amount of the Ackroyds' taxes which may be allocated to welfare state expenditures on this assumption is therefore 69.2% of the total taxes they pay, or £95,523. If this is compared with the value of direct expenditures on the Ackroyds (£154,461), they could be said to receive a 'subsidy' from the welfare state of £58,938.

The Osbornes pay £210,794 in income tax and national insurance contributions (27% of life-time earnings) and £159,198 in other taxes (21% of life-time earnings). The amount of taxes which can be allocated to welfare state expenditures on the same assumption used for the Ackroyd calculation is £256,034. The total direct expenditures on the Osbornes is £216,416 (Stephen in SERPS) or £175,352 (Stephen contracted out). The Osbornes, on this assumption, could therefore be said to 'subsidise' the welfare state by some amount between £59,618 (Stephen in SERPS) and £80,682 (Stephen contracted out).

The tobacco factor

One reason that the welfare state is not more redistributive is what might be called the tobacco factor. The families of most manual workers or unemployed people, like the Ackroyds, contain at least one smoker (Family Expenditure Survey, 1984, cited in Fry and Pashardes, 1988). Smokers make fewer demands of the welfare state. For example, J. Wilkinson (1986, p.80) cites figures indicating that a 20% drop in smoking in 1971 would have saved £4m in health care costs by 1981, but increased social security costs by £12m by the year 2000. Smokers also pay substantial amounts in indirect taxes: tobacco revenue raises some £1b a year (Wilkinson, 1986, p.80); the bottom quintile of non-retired households paid 4.7% of the disposable income in tobacco duty in 1984, while the top quintile paid 1.3% (CSO, 1986a).

These overall trends are reflected in our figures. The demands the Osbornes make on the welfare state in old age, including health care costs as well as retirement pensions, offset the invalidity pension received by Jim Ackroyd. The Ackroyds pay a greater percentage of their life-time earnings in indirect taxes than the Osbornes, reflecting, in part, the fact that low-income families are more likely to smoke.

Summary

Principal conclusions

The principal conclusions are as follows:

1. Some cash benefits, specifically income tested, disability and unemployment related benefits, favour the working class Ackroyds over the middle class Osbornes. Taking all cash benefits except retirement pensions, the Ackroyds receive over four times as much over their life-times as the Osbornes.
2. Retirement pensions on the other hand, benefit the Osbornes more than the Ackroyds. Because they have a longer life expectancy, the Osbornes receive approximately twice as much from the State either directly, if they stay in State Earnings Related Pension Scheme, or indirectly through tax reliefs on private pensions if they contract out.
3. Social services also overwhelmingly favour the middle class Osbornes. Taking housing (including mortgage interest tax relief), health education (including tax subsidies to private education), public transport and the arts together, the Osbornes receive 2.3 times as much. This arises in large part because of their greater life expectancy (leading to greater use of the Health Service), their university education, their use of public transport for commuting and their visits to the subsidised performing arts.
4. The total of cash benefits and direct expenditures on health and education taken together favour the Ackroyds and the Osbornes about equally. However, the inclusion of subsidies to public transport and the arts, and the various tax reliefs (mortgage interest tax relief, etc.) tip the overall total heavily in favour of the Osbornes who receive 40% more than the Ackroyds.
5. If the finance of the welfare state is taken into account, the system as a whole may redistribute income, since taxes bear more heavily on higher income groups. On one assumption concerning the incidence of the taxes that finance welfare, the working class Ackroyds gain £58,938 from the welfare state (direct expenditures net of taxes) while the Osbornes subsidise the welfare state by an amount between £59,618 and £80,682. The financing of the welfare state has, however, become less progressive in recent years.

A concluding comment

Since 1985/86, a number of changes have been made in the tax and social security systems. While these changes are significant, we expect that they would not alter our basic conclusions.

In April, 1988, family income supplement was replaced with family credit, supplementary benefit with income support, and changes were made to the rules governing housing benefit. The changes would not benefit the Ackroyds or the Osbornes. A simulation with the programme TAXBEN (designed by the London School of Economics by A. Atkinson, H. Sutherland, and B. Warren) shows that the Ackroyds would not be eligible for family credit (assuming Jim's income level has risen to £160 per week). Income support replaces grants for furniture and so on with loans, and reduces the number of passport benefits. However, as these benefits were not included in our original calculations, the elimination of these benefits will not affect our results. One change which might work to the detriment of the Ackroyds is the imposition of a capital limit of £8,000, above which housing and other benefits cannot be claimed. This might lower the amount of housing benefit received by the Ackroyds, particularly during retirement.

The 'Fowler reforms' to pensions could reduce the welfare state benefits received by the Osbornes. The reforms to SERPS mean that a person can only inherit half his or her spouse's SERPS entitlement. If Stephen Osborne was in SERPS, this would reduce the amount that Henrietta receives after Stephen's death by £5,138. If, however, Stephen Osborne contracts out, the reforms will have no effect.

A final change is the reduction in tax rates, particularly as the higher income levels. The effect of reduced taxes is to make welfare state finance significantly less redistributive. Table 5 shows the changes in income tax as a percentage of earnings for various income groups. However, as tax rates fall, the value of the tax reliefs claimed by the Osbornes falls also. The net effect of these two trends is difficult to predict.

It is possible that the trend toward less progressive financing of the welfare state will continue. If so, and if the fact that the Osbornes do so much better than the Ackroyds out of key areas of the welfare state is regarded as unjust, the perceived injustices will become yet greater.

NOTE

This paper was the basis for the Granada World in Action programme 'Spongers' broadcast on 15 May 1989. The programme used 1988/89 figures (rather than 1985/86 as here); it also made comparisons with 1978/79. Those estimates can be found in Woolley (1989).

Acknowledgements

This study was commissioned by Granada Television, whose support is gratefully acknowledged. We would also like to acknowledge support received under the ST/ICERD Welfare State Programme and the ESRC, grant number X206322001. We are very grateful to Don Jordan of Granada for constructing the basic life histories of the Ackroyds and the Osbornes, and to John Hills for comments. None of the above are, of course, responsible for any errors in the paper.

Appendix:
Calculation of Benefits

Life expectancies

The 1971 Occupational Mortality Survey estimates that a professional male's life expectancy at 15 is 103% of the average (57.2/55.6), while an unskilled worker's life expectancy is 96% of the average (53.5/55.6). Applying these figures to current life expectancies of 71.4 years for a male, 77.2 for a female (Social Trends, 1986) yields the life expectancies given in the text.

Earnings

Principal source: Department of

TABLE 5
Single earner married couple with two children

Earnings % average	1978/79 %	1987/88 %	Changes as % income
50	2.5	5.9	+3.4
75	14.6	15.9	+1.3
100	20.9	21.0	+0.1
150	26.2	24.8	-1.4
200	27.9	26.4	-5.7

Source: CPAG (1988)

Employment (DE) (1986).

The salary levels are taken from the new Earnings Survey (DE, 1986), which gives the national average wage for each occupational group. Jim Ackroyd earns £150 per week as a fork-lift operator, and £155 as a security guard. This is about 10% less than the national averages of £165 and £169.4 respectively. Stephen Osborne's salary of £350 per week is taken to be closer to that of a finance, insurance, tax etc. specialist (£403.7 per week) than to that of an accountant (£268.7 per week).

Cash benefits

Principal sources: Allbeson and Douglas (1985); DHSS (1986); UK (1985b).

The cash benefits considered here are child benefit, family income supplement, housing benefit, invalidity pension, sickness

TABLE A.1
Benefits by life cycle stage – the Osbornes

Life cycle stage	Duration (years)	Earnings (£p.w.)	Benefits received (£p.w.)
Children are under 18, in full-time education	18	£350	child (£7 per child)
Stephen's illness 3 x eight weeks (two attacks and bypass)	0.46	n/a	statutory sick pay (£44.35)
nine weeks (after bypass)	0.17	n/a	sickness benefit (£29.15)
Other times			none

TABLE A.2
Benefits by life cycle stage – the Ackroyds

Life cycle stage	Duration (years)	Earnings (£p.w.)	Benefits received (£p.w.)
Two children, Jim working, Tracy at home	14	155	child (£7 per child)
Tracy returns to work	2	198	child (£7 per child)
Children looking for work	1a	n/a	supplementary (£18.20)
Whole family is employed	4	198	none
Jim loses his job			
first year	1	43b	unemployment (£30.45)
second year	1	43b	supplementary (£10.85)
			housing benefit (£26)
Jim works as security guard	10	203	none
Jim's emphysema attack			
first eight weeks	0.16	43	statutory sick pay (£30)
			housing benefit (£20)
next 6 months	0.5	43	sickness benefit (£29.15)
			housing benefit (£20)
invalidity pension	5.5	43	invalidity pension (£63.85)
			housing benefit (£7.50)
Tracy's retirement	3.5	nil	invalidity (£63.85)
			housing benefit (£19)
Jim reaches 65	3	nil	retirement pension (£66)
			housing benefit (£19)
Tracy's widowhood	2.6	nil	retirement pension (£41)
			housing benefit (£21)

a Each child spends six months looking for work after leaving the YTS
b Tracy earns £43 per week.
Source: DHSS (1986)

TABLE A.3
Estimate 1 – 'Contracted in' pension benefits 1985/86

	Weekly benefit		Years in receipt		Total	
	Ackroyds	Osbornes	Ackroyds	Osbornes	Ackroyds	Osbornes
	£	£			£	£
Husband's pension						
basic	38,30	38.30				
SERP	3.00	24.70				
graduated	2.07	2.70				
Total	43.37	65.70	3.7	8.4	8,344	28,423
Wife's benefits						
adult dependent	23.00	23.00	3.7	8.4	4,425	10,046
widow's benefit	41.30	63.00	7.6	8.0	16,342	26,208
Total					29,111	64,677

benefit, statutory sick pay, supplementary benefit and unemployment benefit. A number of smaller benefits have been omitted, such as death grant (£30 at death, November 1985) and maternity grant (£25 per child).

Tables A.1 and A.2 show the benefits received by each family in each stage of the life-cycle. It is straightforward to calculate the total amount of benefit once benefit rates are known. Two assumptions were made in arriving at the benefit levels. First, it was assumed that the Ackroyds pay £20.50 in rent and £4.40 in rates per week, which is the average cost of local authority housing for a family with children. (DHSS, 1986). Second, no allowance was made for special grants or passport benefits received while the Ackroyds were on supplementary benefit.

Pensions

Principal sources: DHSS (1986); DHSS (1987); Government Actuary (1985); Papadakis and Taylor-Gooby (1987); UK (1985a); Wilkinson, M. (1986).

Estimate 1: Stephen Osborne and Jim Ackroyd 'contracted in'
– Note on calculation method:

Pensions are calculated so as to correspond to the benefits Jim and Stephen would have received if retiring in 1985. Jim receives a SERP based on his earning in the two years prior to his illness. Stephen receives a SERP based on eight years of contributions prior to his early retirement. Each receives a graduated component based on earning related entitlements acquired prior to 1975.

Benefit levels are taken from DHSS (1986) and DHSS (1987). The SERP entitlement is calculated as one and one quarter per cent of earnings between the upper and lower earnings limits for each year in SERPS. The graduated component is valued at the average amount received by a man aged 65-69 (DHSS, 1986). The SERP entitlement is transferred in full to widows.

Estimate 2: Stephen 'contracted out'
– Calculation of direct expenditures –
the Osbornes:

The effect of contracting out on direct expenditures will be to reduce Stephen's SERP entitlement to nil, and Henrietta's widow's benefit to £38.30 per week. The direct expenditures on the Osbornes' pensions will fall to £43,613.

– Calculation of tax relief – the Osbornes

The cost of tax relief on occupational pensions has two components. The first is tax relief on the lump-sum payment, estimated by Inland Revenue (1983) at £650m. The second is relief on investment income, valued at £2,350m (assuming a 30 per cent tax rate and unchanged employer contributions; Fry, Hammond & Kay, 1985). The two components add up to £3,000m annually. Dividing this sum between the 11.1 million employees in occupational pension schemes in 1983 (Government Actuary, 1985), gives an annual tax expenditure of £270 for an average employee. If Stephen's pension contributions are average, the subsidy over 40 years of employment is £10,810. However, Papadakis and Taylor-Gooby (1987) estimate that a family with income over £350 per week contributes 1.86 times more per week to pension funds and life assurances than does an average family. Using this factor to adjust for contribution size yields an estimate of life-time expenditure of £20,140.

Total indirect expenditures:
– unadjusted – £10,810
– adjusted   – £20,140

Estimate 3: Henrietta 'opting in'
– direct expenditures – the Osbornes:

Henrietta is assumed to receive an own-account pension of £35.40 per week, the average for a woman on her own insurance. The pension received is less than the basic pension as many women do not have enough contributions for full basic pension entitlements (DHSS, 1987).

Total direct expenditures: £26,507

Social Services

Education

Principal sources: Chartered Institute of Public Finance and Accountancy (CIPFA), personal communication (available from authors on request); HM Treasury (1988); DES (1985); University Grants Committee (1987); ISIS (1987), (1988); Papadakis and Taylor-Gooby (1987).

– Direct expenditures

Table A.4 shows the amount of time the children in each family spend in publicly financed education, the cost of schooling and the total expenditure on each child.

– Tax reliefs – the Osbornes:

Tax relief while the Osbornes' children are at private school is calculated by dividing Papadakis and Taylor-Gooby's estimate (1987) of the subsidies to the private sector from tax and rate relief (£42 million in 1986/87) by the ISIS (1987) estimate of the total number of students in independent schools (560,000 students in 1986), producing an estimated subsidy of £75 per pupil

per year, or £600 over eight years. This subsidy compares with mid-range school fees of £4,500 per year (ISIS 1987).

The tax expenditure while the children are in university is assumed to be £1134 per child, obtained through the parents covenanting the mandatory grant of £1,400 to their children (providing the children are 18 or older) and obtaining tax relief at the basic rate (27%).

Total tax relief (2 children): £3470
Direct expenditures and tax relief: £47,146

Health care

Principal sources: HM Treasury (1988); OPCS (1978).

– Direct expenditures:

The health care expenditure figures are based on Treasury estimates of annual NHS expenditures per head by age group (1985/86). An average adult between 16 and 64 costs the NHS £190 per year, while a person 65 or over costs £570 per year. Children (excluding birth costs) cost between £235 and £340 annually (HM Treasury, 1988). Applying these rates to the Ackroyds and the Osbornes reveals that Jim Ackroyd receives expenditures of £17,494 over his life-time, while Tracy receives £20,686. The corresponding figure for Stephen Osborne is £20,686 and for Henrietta Osborne is £23,593. The Osbornes' total benefits are greater, because of their longer life expectancy.

Total direct expenditures:
Ackroyds – £38,180
Osbornes – £43,766

Housing
– the Ackroyds:

For benefit rates see 'Cash Benefits'.

TABLE A.4
Direct education expenditures

	Years spent per child		Annual	Total Expenditure	
	Ackroyds	Osbornes	Cost	Ackroyds	Osbornes
			£	£	£
Nursery	1	1	1,103	1,103	1,103
Primary	7	5	727a, 751b	5,089	3,755
Secondary	5	-	1,081	5,405	-
YTS	0.5	-	2,844	1,422	-
University	-	3	5,660c		16,980
Total:					
one child				12,105	21,838
two children				24,210	43,676

a,b Figures taken for CIPFA, per comm. The higher of the two figures is for the Osbornes.
c Consists of £5,250 (cost of one year of university, given by DES, 1985), plus £410 minimum grant.

– The Osbornes

The Osbornes' before tax mortgage payments are assumed to be £52.47 per week. Basic rate mortgage interest relief is £14.16 per week. Assuming 35 years of mortgage payments, the total tax reliefs received by the Osbornes are £25,763.

Total expenditures: £25,763

Public Transport

Principal sources: HM Treasury (1988).

– The Ackroyds

Jim travels by bus twice a day, five days a week, 45 weeks a year, throughout 31 working years. Each bus journey receives a 9.6 pence subsidy (calculated by dividing local authority revenue support for public transport by the total number of passenger journeys on local bus services in Metropolitan and Shire county areas; HM Treasury, 1988). Making some allowance for travel when Jim is unemployed or semi-retired, the total travel subsidy is £1,580 over the life-time.

Total expenditures: £1,580

– The Osbornes

Stephen Osborne commuted 25 miles from High Wycombe to London five times a week, 45 weeks a year, throughout his working life. The Public Service Obligation subsidy per passenger mile is 4.65 pence (1985.86), implying an annual subsidy of £523. Making some allowance for the Osbornes' children's travel and for Stephen's travel after he retires, the total life-time subsidy is £21,109.

Total expenditures: £21,109.

Subsidies to the arts

Principal sources: OAL (1984), (1987); DE (1987).

– The Osbornes

It is assumed that the Osbornes spend their entire entertainment budget on the theatre, but that they spend the same amount on entertainment as others in their income group. The Family Expenditure Survey (DE, 1987) allows us to calculate the Osbornes' life-time entertainment expenditures as £6,322 or £5,374 net of VAT. For subsidised theatre and opera, earned income constitutes 45% of total income (see OAL (1987) for theatre or OAL (1984) for opera). Box office earnings represent about 75% of total earnings. These figures allow us to infer that the Osbornes' box office spending is matched by a grant of £8,758 over the course of their life-time.

Total expenditures: £8,758

Taxation

Principal sources: CSO (1986a,b); HM Treasury (1988).

Notes on the CSO estimates

The CSO's (1986a,b) estimates of the effects of taxes and benefits on household income are used to calculate the income tax, national insurance contributions, and other taxes paid by the Ackroyds and the Osbornes. There are a number of limitations to the estimates, both in general, and in the specific context of this paper. One general problem is that not all taxes can be allocated to households – for example, employers' national insurance contributions. A second is that the Family Expenditure Survey (DE, 1987), on which the CSO estimates are based, under-reports expenditure on certain commodities, including tobacco and alcohol (Fry and Pashardes, 1988), complicating the estimation of the indirect taxes paid on these commodities. Finally, in the specific context of this paper, the CSO estimates are group averages, and do not represent the expenditures of any family whether typical or atypical.

– Taxes paid – the Ackroyds

The Ackroyds, at each stage in their life, are assumed to pay the same amount of taxes as an average household in their decile of the income distribution. For example, when Jim is working but Tracy is not, the family is in the fifth decile of the income distribution. The CSO (1986a,b) estimate that a household in the fifth decile pays £1,198 in income tax and NIC and £1,860 in other taxes. These figures, and others like them, are used to produce an estimate of the taxes paid by the Ackroyds over their life-times. The Ackroyds, over their life-time, pay £54,135 in income taxes and national insurance contributions, and £83,904 in other taxes. Since their life-time earnings are £286,364, taxes as a percentage of earnings are 19% for income tax and 29% for other taxes.

– Taxes paid – the Osbornes:

The Osbornes' life-time tax bill is estimated the same way as the Ackroyds'. The Osbornes, over their life-time, pay £210,794 in income tax and national insurance contributions, and £159,198 in other taxes. As their life-time earnings amount to £763,658, taxes as a percentage of income are 27% for income tax, and 21% for other taxes.

– Proportion to allocate to welfare state expenditures:

In 1985/86, government expenditures of £92.5 billion went to the welfare state, as defined in this paper, out of a planning total of £133.7 billion. The welfare state thus accounts for 69.2% of government expenditure. The major components of welfare state expenditure were Education and Science (£14.4 billion), health and personal social services (£16.6 billion) and social security (£41.5 billion, England only) (HM Treasury, 1988).

References

Allbeson, J. and Douglas, J. (1985) *National welfare benefits handbook*. London: Child Poverty Action Group.

Atkinson, A. (1985) '*Social insurance and income maintenance: a survey*', London School of Economics: ST/ICERD/Welfare State Programme Discussion paper No. 5.

Central Statistical Office (ISO) (1986a,) '*The effects of taxes and benefits on household income, 1984.*' Economic Trends, 393, 101-116.

Central Statistical Office (1986b) '*The effects of taxes and benefits on household income, 1985.*' Economic Trends, 397, 96-109.

Child Poverty Action Group (CPAG) (1988) *Chance for a change: the 1988 budget and beyond*. London: CPAG Ltd.

Department of Education and Science (DES) (1985) *The development of higher education into the 1990s*. London: HMSO.

Department of Employment (DE)(1986) *New earnings survey, 1986*. London: HMSO.

Department of Employment (1987) *Family expenditure survey, 1986*. London: HMSO.

Department of Health and Social Security (DHSS)(1986) *Social security statistics 1987*. London: HMSO.

Fry, V., Hammon, E. and Kay, J. (1985) *Taxing pensions*. IFS Report Series No. 14. London: Institute for Fiscal Studies.

Fry and Pashardes, P. (1988) *Changing patterns of smoking; are there economic causes?* IFS Report Series No. 30. London: Institute for Fiscal Studies.

Goodin, R. and Le Grand, J. (1987) *Not only the poor: the middle classes and the welfare state*. London: Allen & Unwin.

Government Actuary (1985) *Occupational pension schemes 1983: seventh survey by the Government Actuary*. London: HMSO.

H.M. Treasury (1988) *The government's expenditure plans 1988-89 to 1990-92, CM. 288-11*. London: HMSO.

Independent School Information Service (ISIS)(1987) *Basic facts about independent schools*. London: ISIS.

ISIS (1988) *School fees*, London: ISIS.

Inland Revenue (1983) *Cost of tax reliefs for pension schemes: appropriate statistical approach*. Board of Inland Revenue.

Le Grand, J. (1982) *The strategy of equality*. London: Allen and Unwin.

Office of Arts and Libraries (OAL) (1984) *Financial scrutiny of the Royal Opera House Covent Garden Ltd*. London: HMSO.

Office of Arts and Libraries (1987) *Arts Council Annual report 1986/87*. London: HMSO.

Office of Population Censuses and Survey (OPCS) (1978) *Occupational mortality: the Registrar General's decennial supplement for England and Wales, 1970-1972, Series DS No.1*. London: HMSO.

OPCS (1986) *The general household survey 1984*. London: HMSO.

Oster, G., Colditz, G. and Kelly N. (1984) *The economic costs of smoking and benefits of quitting*. Lexington Mass: Lexington Books.

Papadakis, E. and Taylor-Gooby, P. (1987) *The private provision of public welfare*. Brighton, Sussex: Wheatsheaf Books.

Rawls, J. (1973) *A theory of justice*. Oxford: Oxford University Press.

UK(1985a) *The reform of social security, Vol. 1 Cmnd 9517*. London: HMSO.

UK(1985b) *The reform of social security, Vol. 3: Background papers, Cmnd. 9519*. London: HMSO.

University Grants Committee (1987) *University statistics, 1985/86, Vol. 3*. Cheltenham: Universities Statistical Record.

Wilkinson, J. (1986) *Tobacco: the facts behind the smokecreen*. Harmondsworth, Middlesex, Penguin Books.

Wilkinson, J. (1986) '*Tax expenditures and public expenditure in the UK*', Journal of Social Policy, Vol. 15, 23-49.

Woolley, F. (1989) '*The Ackroyds, the Osbornes, and the welfare state: an addendum*'. London School of Economics: ST/ICERD Welfare State Programme Research Note No. 18.

Who cares about equity in the NHS?

RESOURCE 3

Margaret Whitehead, 'Who cares about equity in the NHS?', British Medical Journal, May 1994

The concept of equity in relation to the National Health Service in Britain encompasses not one but at least eight distinct principles. Until the 1980s the NHS had a good record of incorporating these principles into practice. Throughout the 1980s, however, there has been a pronounced change, with the gradual introduction of business values into the service, culminating in the market based reforms of the 1990s. Several recent policies seem to be taking the NHS away from the goal of an equitable system - for example, the new arrangements for community care and the incentives within contracting to select patients on financial grounds. To restore equity as a value demands priority for ethical values, monitoring of policies for their effects on equity, some national planning, and a new debate about the entitlement to services such as continuing care.

Over the past decade successive reorganisations of the NHS have been presented as technical adjustments, to improve efficiency, quality, and patient choice but without affecting the basic equitable foundations of the service. The impression is of noble intentions, but if we dig beneath the rhetoric is the principle of equity being upheld and protected, or is it being quietly abandoned?

Why the NHS was established

In the midst of continual reorganisation it is easy to forget why the NHS was set up in the first place. The political consensus for change grew out of a widespread realisation that the pre-war system was inequitable, inefficient, and near to financial collapse.[12] In the 1930s, for instance, only 43% of the population were covered by the national insurance scheme, mainly men in manual and low paid occupations and only for general practitioner services.[1] That left 21 million people, predominantly the wives and children of employed men, not covered by the scheme. The sick carried much of the burden of payment and could be faced with a devastating bill.

Across Britain services were spread unevenly, with deprived areas poorly served both in quantity and quality of service. This arose because doctors needed to make a living from private practice and only in more prosperous districts could local authorities raise enough local taxes to provide a range of high quality public services. In some places the same practitioner provided a highly visible two tier service.

> Sometimes middle class patients go to the doctor's front door and working class patients to the surgery door. One class of patient comes by appointment, the other is expected to take his turn and may have a considerable time to wait.[3]

A highly fragmented and unplanned service added to the haphazard and inefficient use of resources.[4] For example, 1000 voluntary hospitals and 2000 municipal hospitals were all administered separately and often competed with one another. In 1945 the National Hospital Survey reported that in some places increasing competition for dwindling charitable donations had led to wasteful duplication of equipment and high technology processes in desperate ploys to attract funds.[5 6] Competing hospitals were also reluctant to transfer fee paying patients to a more suitable hospital because of the loss of revenue.

The basis of a more equitable service

Against this background a wide consensus

formed in the 1940s about the need to build a more equitable service and what the principles and values of such a service should be[1]. The concept of equity in the NHS articulated by Aneurin Bevan, the minister of health responsible for introducing the NHS, and later by the Royal Commission in 1979 [7] was multifaceted, incorporating the following principles:

A service for everyone - Everyone was to be included in the scheme as of right, without having to undergo a means test or any other test of eligibility.

Sharing financial costs and free at the point of use - In the words of Bevan: "It has been the firm conclusion of all parties that money ought not to be permitted to stand in the way of obtaining an efficient health service."[8] The method of funding chosen, through general taxation, was linked to the ability to pay.

Comprehensive in range - There was a clear commitment to extend coverage - to preventive, treatment, and rehabilitation services, covering mental as well as physical health, chronic as well as acute care.

Geographical equality - With the intention of creating "a national service, responsive to local needs,"[7] came a commitment to improve the geographical spread of services.

The same high standard of care for everyone - The Royal Commission emphasised that this principle must be based on levelling up, not levelling down: "The aim must be to raise standards in areas where there are deficiencies but not at the expense of places where services are already good."[7]

Selection on the basis of need for health care, not financial position in situations of scarcity. People had the right to expect that no one would be able to gain access to a service ahead of others, by money or social influence.

The encouragement of a non-exploitative ethos, to be achieved by maintaining high ethical standards and by minimising incentives for making profits from patients. As the Royal Commission noted: "We are well aware that some of these objectives lack precision and some are controversial ... We are aware too that some are unattainable, but that does not make them any less important as objectives."[7]

What progress in putting principles into practice?

Up to the early 1980s deliberate policies were being pursued, with varying degrees of success, to move towards a more equitable service. Throughout the 1980s, however, there has been a sharp change, with the gradual introduction of business values and encouragement of the private sector, culminating in the market based reforms of the 1990s. Butler summarised the four key developments in the 1980s which laid the groundwork for a change of ethos [9]: (a) the introduction of general management from 1984, making the NHS more open to political influence; (b) the introduction of "income generation", releasing previous inhibitions about making profits and engaging in entrepreneurism; (c) the policy of making health authorities contract out some services, establishing the principle that it was not necessary to provide a service, only to commission or "purchase" it; and (d) the international growth of interest in market solutions to cost containment problems.

Working For Patients in 1989 built on these developments to promote the idea of competition and of exposing services to market forces to a much greater degree. But by its nature competition creates winners and losers. If balancing the books becomes the overriding consideration, then it could easily lead to a health service for groups who may have less need but be more lucrative. The losers in health care could be less profitable services, areas of the country, and groups in society. Three examples of progress and retreat on these values may clarify these points.

Entitlement and pooling of financial costs

In 1948 universal entitlement was accomplished at a stroke, as was making services free at the point of use, thus opening up a wide range of services previously out of the financial reach of large sections of the population. The system of funding largely through general taxation has persisted and has recently been assessed as one of the most progressive funding systems among 10 countries in the Organisation for Economic Co-operation and Development. [10] Together these components of the system broke the link between the need for health care and the ability to pay for it - removing the fear of devastating bills. This has been rated as one of the NHS's greatest achievements. [7]

The principle of free treatment at the point of use, however, has been eroded, with the introduction, firstly, of prescription charges in 1951 and later of the charges for dental and ophthalmic services. This policy of charging has continued under both Conservative and Labour governments but has accelerated in the 1980s. For example, the proportion of the total cost of the NHS in the United Kingdom derived from charges (prescriptions, dental fees, and private health care) rose from 2% in 1978-9 to 2.9% in 1984-5 and to 4.5% in 1990.[11] A much higher burden of charges falls on specific services such as dentistry and ophthalmic care (Department of Health, personal communication). The full effect of charging on access to these services is hard to gauge

because it has occurred almost simultaneously with an exodus of opticians and dentists from the NHS.

Continuing care

The most disturbing erosion of the principle of entitlement to a comprehensive range of free services has been in continuing care. The shedding of responsibility for continuing care was made possible by a change in the social security regulations in 1980, allowing social security support to people living in private residential and nursing care. As a result there has been an explosion of such provision, [12] and hard pressed NHS managers have been only too willing to transfer patients into private homes to relieve the NHS budget. The effect, however, has been to switch patients from a free service into a means tested one. Moreover , since 1993 patients have also had to undergo eligibility tests devised by their local authority, which vary across the country.

The evidence of resulting hardship caused to some patients and their relatives is mounting. [13] [14] In a case brought before the health service ombudsman in February 1994 the ombudsman condemned the action of a health authority in transferring a stroke victim to a nursing home for which his family had to find £6000 in top up fees. This brings back the spectre of devastating bills for health care. It also raises the likelihood of an expansion of the gradual transfer of free NHS services into means tested services, particularly in the non-acute and community health sectors.

Levelling up the standard of care around the country

When the NHS came into being it inherited such enormous inequalities in the pattern and quality of services around the country that a clutch of major policy initiatives was required to tackle the issue.

The hospital plan

From the earliest days the redeployment of hospital staff around the country, made possible by having a unified service with salaried staff on national pay scales, resulted in an immediate increase in the number of specialists, junior medical staff, and nurses in poorly served areas of Britain. [4] In 1962 the hospital plan represented the first attempt in Western Europe to plan a hospital building programme strategically to improve access for the population in each region. Much of the building work was completed, providing new district general hospitals in many parts of the country, but the programme ran out of steam when the money dried up in the 1970s.

Primary care

In primary care the distribution of general practitioners was dramatically improved in the early years by the dual strategies of negative control (prohibiting new practices in well provided areas) and financial incentives (allowances for setting up in underdoctored areas), but progress had slowed by the 1960s. An increase in the total number of general practitioners in the 1970s produced a further decline in the number of underdoctored areas. [15] In 1952 more than half the population of England and Wales lived in underdoctored areas, whereas by 1980 the figure was down to 5% per cent and has continued to improve. [16] There was still, however, a serious quality divide between services in deprived and affluent areas reported in 1989. [17]

Resource allocation formulas

The introduction in 1976 of a national resource allocation formula (RAWP) was the first concerted attempt to base resource allocation for hospital and community health services on the need for health care rather than on the historical pattern of services. A standardised mortality ratio was used as a proxy for need, the formula favoured the relatively poorer regions of Britain, with their higher mortality rates. [18] In 1976 the expenditure per head of population in the wealthiest regions was about 30% higher than that of the poorest regions. After a decade of the RAWP formula the gap had fallen to less than 10%. [19] In that respect the formula succeeded in reducing regional inequalities but as it was applied at a time of severe financial restriction, the reduction was achieved by cutting the resources to the wealthiest regions at the same time as improving those to the poorest.

Region	% Change in funding
Northern	-1.3
Yorkshire	-0.6
Trent	-0.8
East Anglia	-0.1
North West Thames	1.9
Norh East Thames	0.8
South East Thames	1.1
South West Thames	1.6
Wessex	2.8
Oxford	0.1
South Western	1.9
West Midlands	-1.7
Mersey	-1.1
North Western	-2.6

Change in regional target funding by applying reduced weighting to standardised mortality ratios in capitation based formula (1988-9 figures)

More recent policies

All these policies represented serious attempts to tackle geographical inequalities in health care, a commitment which seems to be lacking in more recent policies. For example, by reducing the weighting given to standardised mortality the new capitation formula introduced in 1991 has channelled resources away from the less affluent regions with high premature mortality, mainly in the north, towards those with lower premature mortality, mainly in the south and east (table). [20] Regions have been encouraged to use the same formula for subregional allocations, but again the effect has been to shift resources away from some deprived inner city districts with high mortality and morbidity to more prosperous, healthier districts. [21] Such attempts have been abandoned in some areas in favour of approaches which recognise areas that are poorly served and with poorer health profiles. A revised national formula is expected any day, based on 1991 census data, but it is not clear that it will be based on principles more equitable than those in the previous version.

In primary care, the general practitioners' contract of 1990 and the fundholding scheme started in 1991 look set to widen, rather than narrow, the quality divide in general practice. No national pattern has emerged, but initial reports suggest that in some regions uptake of fundholding, attracting associated resources, was strongest among the better resourced practices in more prosperous areas. [22] [23] Likewise, the financial incentives to develop new services for patients under the general practitioner contract have proved easier to achieve in middle class areas as many depend on achieving targets for uptake of a service, which both are easier to achieve in middle class areas and swell the flow of resources to these areas. [24]

To this list can be added the effect of new funding arrangements for community care, which seem to reinforce existing inequalities in provision, draining resources from inner city areas into more prosperous seaside locations.[25] None of these developments suggest that the principle of planning for equitable geographical distribution of services is being addressed seriously. Moreover, the fragmentation of the service into many separate competing units will damage the ability to plan strategically still further.

Selection on financial grounds

With much of the NHS based on salaried service, minimal fees for service arrangements, and limited private insurance coverage, until about 1980 there was little opportunity to select patients on financial grounds. Although primary and community health services and emergency secondary care scored well on this principle, queue jumping for elective surgery has always been possible, with NHS consultants allowed to have a private practice alongside their NHS work. From indirect evidence on consultants' contracts however, the opportunity for queue jumping was probably of minor importance until the beginning of the 1980s.

Consultants' contracts were then relaxed and private health insurance encouraged. Since then there has been a steady increase in commercial medicine, particularly in London, where in 1989-90 NHS consultants as a body were earning more in private fees than from the NHS. [26]

This mixing of NHS and private work has raised questions about both equity and the efficient running of NHS Hospitals. [26]

With the introduction of the Working for Patients reforms in 1991 increased opportunities to select patients on financial grounds have emerged. Some fundholders have achieved improved waiting times for their patients, attention from senior specialists, quicker response times for diagnostic tests, and other improvements. [27] Supporters of the scheme argue that these improvements reflect more efficient purchasing by fundholders than by district purchasers, whereas others suggest that fundholders have been more generously funded. At least one district authority has shown that fundholders within its boundaries were more generously funded than the authority itself and that this coincided with a reduction in waiting lists for fundholders' patients and an increase in those for other patients (see subsequent paper in this series by Dixon [28]).

Surveys by the BMA and the royal colleges have shown that many hospitals are routinely "fast tracking" - giving preference to the patients of fundholders. [29] [30] No one knows quite how widespread these practices are but they pose a threat to the principle of selection on the basis of need, not ability to pay.

This in turn raises the question of what is happening to the ethos of the service. In the past the NHS workforce earned an international reputation for their integrity and altruism. [31] [32] How much the business culture of the 1980s has dented that reputation, or has led to exploitation of the workforce itself, is an aspect that has been neglected by research. There is a danger that the current low morale of health workers and commercial practices such as silencing of criticism, increasing use of short term contracts, and pressure to abandon the values that have inhibited the exploitation of patients for profit may have damaged the fragile ethos of public service.

Prospects for the future

The situation is not without hope. Many working within the NHS are determined to maintain an equitable service, and the public at large wants this principle retained. Much more active promotion of the basic principles needs to be attempted, and here four broad areas of action are suggested.

Return to ethical values

The issue of selection on the basis of financial grounds has to be tackled as a matter of priority and requires a two pronged attack. Firstly, it needs the promotion of ethical values at all levels, not just for individual health professionals but also for managers, administrators, and policymakers in both purchasing and provider authorities. This will not be taken seriously unless the government stops sending mixed messages on the subject - one day issuing guidelines against setting preferential terms in contracts and the next defending fast tracking.

Secondly, organisational changes need to be made to cut out the opportunities to select on financial grounds, thus removing the ethical dilemma. This would involve, for example, devising more equitable methods of resource allocation in health and social care, reducing any built in bias against more deprived areas and groups.

Equity audit

Policymakers need to audit how existing provision and proposed developments affect the provision of an equitable service. Careful monitoring needs to take place of how health status, health hazards, and health and social services are distributed across a given population. Purchasers could do worse than start by asking such questions as, Who gets what services and where? What is known about whether resources are being channelled towards areas of greater need or vice versa? The aim would be to ensure that the flow of resources and the thrust of any targets set went in the right direction, tackling rather than exacerbating current inequalities.

National planning and assessing effectiveness

National planning is required to counteract the tendency towards wasteful duplication and over-treatment generated by competition or the sheer haphazard pattern that emerges from a fragmented system. There also needs to be strict control over the proliferation of untested high technology innovations and much more evaluation of the effectiveness of new service or managerial configurations emerging as a result of the reforms. The continuing collection of comprehensive national statistics needs to be developed and maintained.

A new debate on entitlement

What is happening with continuing care is disturbing and cannot be left to drift into policymaking by default, especially with an ageing population. Should those in need of continuing nursing care no longer be entitled to free NHS services and have to bear the burden of payment or be means tested? There are searching questions to be asked about the long term consequences of excluding some of the most vulnerable members of society from coverage by the NHS. What are the alternatives? Are there other service priorities which are less important? All the options need to be investigated and an equitable solution sought.

References

1   Webster C. *The history of the NHS.* Vol. 1. *Problems of health care.* London HMSO, 1988.

2   Klein R. *The politics of the national Health Service.* London: Longman, 1989.

3   Political and Economic Planning. *The British health service.* London: Political and Economic Planning, 1937.

4   Godber G. *The health service: past, present and future.* London: Athlone Press, 1975.

5   Parsons LG. *Ministry of Health hospital survey: hospital services of the Sheffield and East Midlands area.* London: HMSO, 1945.

6   Gray A, Topping A. *Ministry of Health hospital survey: hospital services of London and surrounding area.* London: HMSO, 1945.

7   Merrison A (chairman). *Report of the Royal Commission on the national Health Service,* London: HMSO, 1979.

8   Bevan A. *Hansard* 30 April 1946.

9   Butler J. Origins and early development In: Robinson R, Le Grand J. (eds) *Evaluating the NHS reforms.* London: King's Fund Institute 1994.

10   van Dooslaer E, Wagstaff A, Rutten F. *Equity in the finance and delivery of health care: an international perspective.* Oxford: Oxford University Press, 1993.

11   Calman M, Cant S, Gabe J. *Going private: why people pay for their medical care.* Buckingham: Open University Press, 1993.

12   House of Commons Health Committee. *Community care: funding from 1993. Third report session 1992/93, House of Commons Papers.* London: HMSO, 1993:309-10.

13   Association of CHCs for England and Wales. NHS continuing care of elderly people. London: ACHCEW, 1990.

14   House of Commons Social Security Committee. *The financing of private residential and nursing home fees. Fourth Report.* London: HMSO, 1991.

15   Butler J, Knight R. *Designated areas: a review of problems and policies.* BMJ 1975; ii:571-3.

16   Derived from *Compendium of health statistics: 8th ed.* London: Office of Health Economics, 1992: table 4.13.

17   Pringle M.*The quality divide in primary care: set to widen under the new contract.* BMJ 1989; 299:470-1.

18   Sheldon T, Davey Smith G, Bevan G. *Weighting in the dare: resource allocation in the new NHS.* BMJ 1993; 306: 835-9.

19   Holland W. W. *The RAWP review: pious hopes.* Lancet 1986;ii:1089-90.

20   Royston G, Hurst J, Lister E, Stewart P. *Modelling the use of health services by population of small areas to inform the allocation of central resources to larger regions.* Socio-economic Planning Science 1992;26:169-80.

21   Moore W. *Cash allocation formula is "unfair" to socially deprived districts.* Health Service Journal 1992;5 Mar:6.

22   Coulter A, Bradlow J. *Effect of NHS reforms on general practitioners' referral patterns.* BMJ 1993;306:433-7.

23   Glennerster H, Matsaganis M, Owens P. *A foothold for fundholding.* London: King's Fund Institute, 1992.

24   Gillam S. *Provision of health promotion clinics in relation to population need: another example of the inverse care law.* Br J Gen Pract 1992;42:54-6.

25   House of Commons. *Local government finances.* Hansard 1993; 11 Feb.

26   Laing W. *Going private: independent health care in London.* London: King's Fund London Initiative, 1992

27   Beecham L. *Fundholders' patients are treated quicker, say BMA.* BMJ 1994; 308:11.

28   Dixon J, Dinwoodie H, Hodson D, Dodd S, Poltorak T, Garrett C, *et al. Are fundholding practices funded more generously than non fundholding practices.* BMJ (in press).

29   *President's letter to fellows and members.* London: RCOG, 1994.

30   Royal College of Surgeons of England. *College survey of surgical activity in the National Health Service.* London RCS, 1994.

31   Schwartz W, Aaron H. *Rationing hospital care: lessons from Britain.* N Engl J Med 1984;310:52.6.

32   Light D. Bending the rules. *Health Service Journal* 1990;100:1513-5.

The targets in full

RESOURCE 4

*Department of Health,
The Health of the Nation
and You, 1992*

Coronary heart disease (CHD) and stroke

To reduce death rates for both CHD and stroke in people under 65 by at least 40% by the year 2000 (from 58 per 100,000 population in 1990 to no more than 35 per 100,000 for CHD and from 12.5 per 100,000 population in 1990 to no more than 7.5 per 100,000 for stroke).

To reduce the death rate for CHD in people aged 65-74 by at least 30% by the year 2000 (from 899 per 100,000 population in 1990 to no more than 629 per 100,000).

To reduce the death rate for stroke in people aged 65-74 by at least 40% by the year 2000 (from 265 per 100,000 population in 1990 to no more than 159 per 100,000).

To reduce the prevalence of cigarette smoking in men and women aged 16 and over to no more than 20% by the year 2000 (a reduction of at least 35% in men and 29% in women, from a prevalence in 1990 of 31% and 28% respectively).

To reduce mean systolic blood pressure in the adult population by at least 5mm Hg by 2005.

To reduce the percentages of men and women aged 16-64 who are obese, by at least 25% for men and at least 33% for women by 2005 (from 8% for men and 12% for women in 1986/87 to no more than 6% and 8% respectively).

To reduce the average percentage of food energy derived by the population from saturated fatty acids by at least 35% by 2005 (from 17% in 1990 to no more than 11%).

To reduce the average percentage of food energy derived by the population from total fat by at least 12% by 2005 (from about 40% in 1990 to no more than 35%).

To reduce the proportion of men drinking more than 21 units of alcohol per week from 28% in 1990 to 18% by 2005 and the proportion of women drinking more than 14 units of alcohol per week from 11% in 1990 to 7% by 2005.

Cancers

To reduce the death rate for breast cancer in the population invited for screening by at least 25% by the year 2000 (from 95.1 per 100,000 population in 1990 to no more than 71.3 per 100,000).

To reduce the incidence of invasive cervical cancer by at least 20% by the year 2000 (from 15 per 100,000 population in 1986 to no more than 12 per 100,000).

To halt the year-on-year increase in the incidence of skin cancer by 2005.

To reduce the death rate for lung cancer by at least 30% in men under 75 and 15% in women under 75 by 2010 (from 60 per 100,000 for men and 24.1 per 100,000 for women in 1990 to no more than 42 and 20.5 respectively).

To reduce the prevalence of cigarette smoking in men and women aged 16 and over to no more than 20% by the year 2000 (a reduction of at least 35% in men and 29% in women, from a prevalence in 1990 of 31% and 28% respectively).

In addition to the overall reduction in prevalence, at least a third of women smokers to stop smoking at the start of their pregnancy by the year 2000.

To reduce the consumption of cigarettes by at least 40% by the year 2000 (from 98 billion manufactured cigarettes per year in 1990 to 59 bn).

To reduce the smoking prevalence among 11-15 year olds by at least 33% by 1994 (from about 8% in 1988 to less than 6%).

Mental illness

To improve significantly the health and social functioning of mentally ill people.

To reduce the overall suicide rate by at least 15% by the year 2000 (from 11.1 per 100,000 population in 1990 to no more than 9.4).

To reduce the suicide rate of severely mentally ill people by at least 33% by the year 2000 (from the estimate of 15% in 1990 to no more than 10%).

Accidents

To reduce the death rate for accidents among children aged under 15 by at least 33% by 2005 (from 6.7 per 100,000 population in 1990 to no more than 4.5 per 100,000).

To reduce the death rate for accidents among young people aged 15-24 by at least 25% by 2005 (from 23.2 per 100,000 population in 1990 to no more than 17.4 per 100,000).

To reduce the death rate for accidents among people aged 65 and over by at least 33% by 2005 (from 56.7 per 100,000 population in 1990 to no more than 38 per 100,000).

HIV/AIDS and sexual health

To reduce the incidence of gonorrhoea among men and women aged 15-64 by at least 20% by 1995 (from 61 new cases per 100,000 population in 1990 to no more than 49 new cases per 100,000).

To reduce the percentage of injecting drug misusers who report sharing injecting equipment in the previous four weeks by at least 50% by 1997, and by at least a further

50% by the year 2000 (from 20% in 1990 to no more than 10% by 1997 and no more than 5% by the year 2000).

To reduce the rate of conception amongst the under 16s by at least 50% by the year 2000 (from 9.5 per 1,000 girls aged 13-15 in 1989 to no more than 4.8).

RESOURCE 5

Department of Health, The Health of the Nation: A Strategy for Health in England, HMSO, 1992

Making the strategy work

The Government's role in developing the strategy – Ministerial Cabinet Committee on Health Strategy – Policy development – Individual opportunities – Healthy alliances – Settings for action – Healthy cities, healthy schools, healthy hospitals, healthy homes, healthy workplaces – Healthy environments – the special role of health professionals.

3.1 The five Key Areas and their targets set out in the previous chapter are at the centre of the strategy for health. The action needed to reach the targets in each of the Key Areas is set out in the appendix.

3.2 Progress towards the targets will also require action across Key Areas. This chapter identifies those who have leading roles within and across Key Areas. It highlights, in particular, the significant opportunities offered by joint working and focusing action on various 'settings' – the home, the school, the workplace, cities and the general environment. It also sets out how Government will support and assist these activities and the general development of the strategy.

Developing the strategy – the Government's role

3.3 The Government is responsible for many elements vital to ensure a healthy population. These responsibilities take a number of forms, including:
  – legislation and regulation
  – providing reliable information on which individuals can base their decisions on matters which affect their health
  – facilitating and encouraging action
  – allocating resources
  – monitoring and assessing changes in health.

3.4 One of the most important tasks of Government is to ensure that Departments work together towards common objectives. The importance Government attaches to this is demonstrated by the establishment of a Ministerial Cabinet Committee to oversee implementation, monitoring and development of the English strat-

egy; and to be responsible for ensuring proper co-ordination of UK-wide issues affecting health.

3.5 Membership of the committee covers 11 Government Departments and it complements existing groups on specific issues such as drugs, alcohol and AIDS.

3.6 The Ministerial Committee will continue to be supported in its work in England by the three Working Groups which were set up following publication of "The Health of the Nation" Green Paper to help with specific aspects of developing and implementing the strategy. These Groups are:
  – a "Wider Health Working Group", chaired by the Minister for Health
  – a "Health Priorities Working Group", chaired by the Government's Chief Medical Officer
  – a "Working Group on Implementation in the NHS", chaired by the Chief Executive of the NHS Management Executive.

Developing policy

3.7 Many policies have, to a greater or lesser degree, an impact on health. It is important, therefore, that as policy is developed the consequences for health are assessed and, where appropriate, taken into account. The Government will produce guidance on 'policy appraisal and health' – a similar approach to the guidance on 'policy appraisal and the environment' which was produced following publication of the Environment White Paper "This Common Inheritance".

Individual opportunities and healthy alliances

3.8 Everyone has a part to play in improving health, and achieving the targets set out in chapter 2. To seize the opportunity, people need information to help make the right choices. Reliable health education in its widest sense is essential for this – pervading education at school and also the many sources of information for people generally about health and its determinants.

3.9 Often the impact on health can be much greater when individuals and organisations work together. Such "healthy alliances" offer a way forward at both local and national level. This approach commanded widespread support during consultation on "The Health of the Nation" Green Paper and many of those responding asked for guidance on forming such healthy alliances. The Department of Health, with the Wider Health Working Group, will prepare and consult on guidance about the promotion of healthy alliances.

The NHS

3.10 One of the key themes of "The Health of the Nation" initiative is that responsibilities for achieving the strategy's objectives and targets go wider than the NHS. Nevertheless, the NHS role as the main provider of health care is crucial to their success. The NHS will need to work with others to initiate and develop common strategies and targets, and to form the healthy alliances needed to take forward action in the Key Areas and other local priorities. The Government looks especially to Regional Health Authorities, working in conjunction with their local health authorities, to initiate the discussion and development of multi-agency approaches to the priorities in this White Paper. The central role of the NHS in the strategy is described more fully in chapter 4.

Local authorities

3.11 Local authorities have an important role in promoting public health and are key players with health authorities in taking forward the policies in this White Paper. In this context they have two principal responsibilities. They are responsible for protecting the environment in which people live and work. They are also responsible for the purchasing and direct provision of social services to meet the needs of the individual members of the public who live in their area. Environmental Health Departments have a special part to play with their responsibilities for health and safety at work, for food safety and food quality, and in collaboration with health authorities for health promotion and investigating and bringing under control outbreaks of communicable disease. Other environmental regulators, Her Majesty's Inspectorate of Pollution and the Drinking Water Inspectorate, will also have an important role.

3.12 As a result of the NHS reforms and the NHS and Community Care Act local authorities, Family Health Services Authorities and District Health Authorities are working with other agencies to look at the needs of the local population and to match their strategies and policies to those local needs. This is leading both to a greater collaboration than before and joint arrangements about the provision of services across agencies.

3.13 Any of these responsibilities on their own would make the input of local authorities to the strategy for health significant. Taken together the contribution of local authorities is vital. Also, with NHS authorities and others in the community, they can take part in local alliances which can develop initiatives to improve the health of local populations.

The health education authority

3.14 The Health Education Authority (HEA) has well-established national programmes of public health education. It also provides a national stimulus to a wide range of local activity. It works, and will continue to work, closely with the media in delivering accurate health education messages, and with the NHS in developing the health promotion and disease prevention roles of the health service. The HEA will be reviewing its strategic aims and objectives in the light of the priorities and targets in this White Paper.

Voluntary organisations

3.15 Voluntary organisations are in a strong position to enhance the health of the population. Between them they cover a broad range of health-related activity. They also have well developed and wide-ranging contracts in, for example, social welfare, sport and recreation, and the environment. More specific roles include:
- through self-help, bringing people together to share common problems and to help them gain more confidence and control over their own health;
- by direct service provision – voluntary organisations have pioneered a wide variety of services;
- in community health, where voluntary organisations work with local people to identify and solve problems affecting their health;
- health education and promotion, education for health professionals, fund raising and support for research.

3.16 The Department of Health supports voluntary organisations engaged in health and personal social services work. Funding in 1992/93 is expected to be of the order of £50 million. Much of the work is already concerned with issues set out in this White Paper. Provision for the largest element of the programme – grants under Section 64 (of the Health Services and Public Health Act 1968) General Scheme – has risen from £15.8 million in 1991/92 to £17.8 million in 1992/93, an increase of 12.5%. The Department of Health has allocated £250,000 in 1992/93 from this increase to fund preliminary voluntary sector work in support of "The Health of the Nation" initiative.

The media

3.17 The media have an important role to play in providing individuals with the information necessary to make decisions which affect their own health and that of their families. People are often confused by the wide variety of sometimes conflicting advice they receive on health matters. It is important therefore that the health messages which people receive from newspapers, magazines, television and radio are accurate, consistent and clear. The Government and the Health Education Authority will play their part by continuing to provide clear and authoritative advice on the factors which can influence health, and on the steps which individuals can take to protect and improve their health.

The workplace

3.18 During their working lives, most people spend around a quarter of their time at work. Employers have long been required to provide safe and healthy working conditions. Increasingly they are also recognising the benefits of a workforce with good general health, while trades unions and staff associations are looking for ways to improve the health of their members. The success of the workplace initiative in the Department of Health/Health Education Authority's 'Look After Your Heart' programme demonstrates this growing demand for advice on health and healthy lifestyles. In four years it has been taken up by more than 500 employers covering 3.8 million employees.

Action in different settings

3.19 "Healthy alliances", either within individual Key Areas or across a number of them, add significantly to the opportunities for progress towards the national targets. Opportunities to work towards the achievement of the targets, and indeed of other health gains, will be similarly enhanced if action – above all joint action – is pursued in various discrete "settings" in the places where people live and work. Such settings include:
–   healthy cities
–   healthy schools
–   healthy hospitals
–   healthy workplaces
–   healthy homes
–   healthy environments
They offer between them the potential to involve most people in the country.

Healthy cities

3.20 A number of cities in England are involved in the WHO 'Healthy Cities' programme. This programme, which started in 1986, now involves 34 European project cities. It seeks to make maximum use of local initiative. Some 75 other towns and cities in England are also involved through the UK Health For All Network, – one of 17 such networks throughout Europe. The UK Health For All Network, based in Liverpool, has been supported by the Health Education Authority. The Government is anxious that the Network continues to provide a means of exchanging information amongst participating towns and cities in England and, through WHO, into the wider European network. The Government will examine ways in which the UK Health For All Network can be further assisted to carry out this work and to increase the number of localities – rural as well as urban – taking part.

3.21 The Government's action to improve housing recognises the broad link between decent local environment and housing conditions and good health. Housing Action Trusts, Estate Action and the Urban Programme are all designed to promote urban renewal, while City Challenge has stimulated proposals from the competing local authorities to make particularly deprived areas more attractive and healthier places in which to live and work. Alongside this, improvements in local health also depend on local initiative to produce a local equivalent of the national strategy for health – highlighting local health issues and seeking to promote health by involving the people and organisations most directly affected.

Healthy schools

3.22 An initiative on healthy schools is being developed jointly by WHO, the European Community and the Council of Europe. This will offer opportunities to reach pupils, parents, staff and all who are associated with schools and education. The Government intends that England should play its full part in this initiative and its development. The Government will seek to establish, jointly with the Health Education Authority and in co-operation with European partners, a pilot network of health promoting schools. This will develop, and assess the effectiveness of, strategies for changing and shaping pupils' patterns of behaviour, with the aim of safeguarding their long-term good health.

Healthy hospitals

3.23 Hospitals exist to provide treatment and care but they also offer unique opportunities for more general health promotion for patients, staff and all who come into contact with them. WHO is currently developing a health promoting hospital initiative. The Government will help with the development of this initiative. The NHS Management Executive will examine how best the concept of health promoting hospitals can be developed and taken forward from the point of view of patients, public and staff.

Healthy workplaces

3.24 The increasing concern of employers and their workforces to improve health opens major opportunities to develop and increase activity on general health promotion in the workplace. This has the advantage of covering all of the key areas. The government will set up a task force to examine and develop activity on health promotion in the workplace. The departments of health and employment, the health and safety executive, the health education authority, representatives from the wider health working group, the confederation of British industry, the trades union congress and other business organisations will be invited to join. The objective will be to advise on new initiatives, including health promotion campaigns and on materials which can be produced for the workplace.

Healthy homes

3.25 The home environment affects many aspects of lifestyle and can have other important effects on health, for example, accidents. For some groups, such as children, parents, people not in outside employment and retired people, it is particularly important. Health professionals, particularly health visitors who work with families in their homes, and general practitioners have a major role in providing information and help so that people based at home can secure healthier ways of life for themselves and for members of their families.

3.26 Good housing is important to good health, although the interdependence between factors such as occupational class, income, unemployment, housing and lifestyle makes it difficult to assess which health effects are specifically attributable to it. The Government's objective is to ensure that decent housing is within the reach of all families. The Government will continue to pursue its policies to promote choice and quality in housing, having regard to health and other benefits.

Healthy prisons

3.27 In May 1992, the former Prison Medical Service was relaunched as the Health Care Service for Prisoners. This change of name signals a clear and increased commitment to health promotion, prevention of ill-health, and treatment. Major developments in Health care for prisoners include:
- the establishment of a Health Advisory Committee, to advise on matters affecting the health of prisoners;
- the development of health standards in the prison setting;
- the development of an effective purchasing role through contracts with the NHS and other providers of clinical services.

Healthy environments

3.28 The quality of the environment is also an important influence on health. The Government White Paper "This Common Inheritance" set out the current targets for improving air and water quality and other environmental objectives which should, amongst other things, help to reduce risk factors to health. The next annual report on the environment later this year will update these targets, and will give particular attention to strengthening the links between environmental objectives and their health consequences. Areas for attention will include:
- air quality standards': An Expert Panel on Air Quality Standards (EPAQS) has been set up to advise

on standards and this panel will be supported by the Committee on the Medical Effects of Air Pollutants. Standards will be set or strengthened for concentrations of sulphur dioxide, ground level ozone, benzene, carbon monoxide, 1:3 butadiene and acid aerosols.

- indoor air quality: Studies of the health effects of various indoor air pollutants including radon, volatile organic compounds, formaldehyde, nitrogen dioxide, mould spores and dust house mites are in hand. Advice on dealing with high levels of radon in homes is already available, with grants for remedial work in some cases. Guidance and other action on other contaminants will be developed as necessary.

- drinking water: Ninety-nine per cent of the tests carried out on drinking water show compliance with regulatory standards. Quality is thoroughly audited by the Chief Drinking Water Inspector. Action to deal with remaining problems is in hand and will be extended, for example to deal with lead contamination in some areas.

- exposure to UV radiation: International action is in hand to eliminate as soon as possible the production of CFCs and other substances which are damaging the ozone layer. A target for skin cancer is set in this White Paper (see appendix B.13).

3.29 Often the most urgent priority is for research to pin-point more accurately the linkage between the quality of the environment and the health consequences. Having in mind the difficulty of establishing these linkages, the Government will explore the advantages of creating a new focus for work on environment and health in the form of a possible new Institute for the Environment and Health. Its work might cover risks to both human health and the natural environment from exposure to hazardous chemicals in the environment (already the National Radiological Protection Board has a similar responsibility for radiation hazards, and the Public Health Laboratory Service for microbiology). At present a variety of Government Departments and other public bodies share interests in this area, and improved co-ordination of work would ensure that effective pro-

grammes could be set up to address the most urgent problems.

The special role of health professionals

3.30 The role of the health professions – and indeed everyone who provides health care and related services – will be crucial to the success of the strategy. The opportunities to help and advise individuals, families and communities are unparalleled.

3.31 The development and adoption of agreed standards of good practice is particularly important. The recent developments in clinical audit are to be commended and should be built on. Leadership in the development of good practice lies primarily with the health professions, and where appropriate, the voluntary sector.

3.32 The Government is keen to explore with professional, voluntary and other bodies opportunities for development and dissemination of standards of good practice, especially where this developed collaboratively. The Government's Chief Professional Officers will discuss with the health professions how further development of standards of good practice and clinical protocols can be taken forward. The Government will also use new and existing machinery, such as the tripartite Task Group it has set up jointly with the General Medical Services Committee and the Royal College of General Practitioners to consider the identification and dissemination of good practice in health promotion for GPs.

3.33 The Department of Health will be exploring ways of creating national and local networks to draw together the scarce public health skills and widespread specialist knowledge needed to take the strategy for health forward.

Professional education and training

3.34 For any strategy to be successful it must be backed by appropriate initial and continuing education and training for all those whose work will be affected by the policies set out in this White Paper. For example, students in medical and dental undergraduate training need to appreciate that disease prevention and health promotion are as important as disease management and the provision of high quality care when considering the overall health of the population. The Government will discuss the need for further emphasis on training in disease prevention and health promotion with the General Medical and Dental

Councils who regulate the under-graduate curriculum and with the Royal College and other bodies who have a key role in postgraduate and continuing medical education.

3.35 In nurse education, Project 2000 is based on a health model which places emphasis on health promotion and disease prevention. The United Kingdom Central Council for Nursing, Midwifery and Health Visiting has consulted widely with the nursing professions on proposals for linking three-yearly re-registration with evidence of continuing education and training.

3.36 Similarly in pharmacy, changes in the degree course over recent years have reflected the changing role of the pharmacist and provide a new emphasis on health promotion and the provision of advice. The same issues will of course, apply to those many other professions involved in health services in the widest sense.

The international dimension

3.37 A successful health strategy cannot be insular. Threats to health may come just as easily from outside the United Kingdom as from within. Collaboration at international level encourages and facilitates the sharing of knowledge and research. Such collaboration in the past has led to the eradication of diseases such as smallpox: it is central to current work on HIV/AIDS. It ensures both a swifter identification of problems and solutions and the most economical use of scarce resources and skills.

3.38 The United Kingdom was a founder member of the World Health Organization. Membership of the European Community and inter-Governmental co-operation on health matters adds a further and specific dimension. The Government will build on these international links to bring the maximum benefit to the nation's health.

Getting the social and health care you need

RESOURCE 6

'Take Care', a series on care in the community, 'You and Yours', BBC Radio 4, April–May 1991

1 Introduction

This factsheet has been designed to help you identify what help and services you might want or need and where you might go locally to find out what services are available and to get help and support. You may be a person in need of help, care and support living on your own or in someone else's home. Or you may be a relative or friend helping to look after somebody else. You may be looking for light domestic help one or two hours per week, or 24 hour a day care. You may be a carer looking for help to let you take regular breaks or to go on holiday.

Everyone has very different needs for community care services. Good community care should be flexible, and responsive to the needs of the carer and the person needing care. The reality in most people's experience is that it is tremendously difficult to find out what services are available or even to know where to go. Most people are used to getting little or no help from statutory or voluntary services which means that expectations are very low. Implementation of the NHS and Community Care Act between now and April 1993 should make some significant improvements to the quantity and quality of information that is available locally about services, particularly because every social services department has to prepare and publish a plan setting out what they will be providing. At the same time the range and type of services provided may also improve – service users and carers should be consulted fully in the planning process and services should reflect and be responsive to their needs and choices.

2 Finding Out

First get in touch with your local social services department or your family doctor. Your local social services department should be able to advise you about the help which it may provide or know about. A social worker should be an important first port of call – they can be the key to getting a service or simply finding out what is available or tell you what might be available from social security benefits. Social services departments are obliged, under the terms of the 1986 Disabled Person's Act, to assess the needs for day services and services at home of people who are disabled. Social services departments have the lead responsibility for community care and, from April 1993, a duty to assess individuals' needs for care and support.

Other places to make a start, or to find out how to contact social services, are advice centres, like Citizens Advice Bureaux, community advice centres and community groups, local Age Concern or Mind groups. A list of useful organisations which produce information, give advice or have local groups or branches, is given at the end of this fact-sheet.

3 What To Ask For

Knowing just what to ask for is also a problem for many people. What is available in your area, will vary – all social services departments offer different kinds of help and will have their own way of deciding who gets what. The numbers and different types of voluntary organisations providing services in your area will also be different.

Work out what you need and how you would like it provided. Some of the services which might be available in your area are listed below. Ask about eligibility criteria, waiting lists, the times at which services are provided and what charges will be made and how frequently these are revised. Some of the things and services that might help you are the following:

Aids, Adaptations and Equipment

Special equipment, gadgets and furniture are available to help with things like turning on taps, getting in and out of bed, moving around, and bathing. Very often a rail near the bath or sink can be very helpful. Adaptations to your home can include ramps, widening doors, lifts. Get advice from an occupational therapist who may also supply equipment, and aids will come from the National Health Service, via hospitals or community nurses, some from social services and some from GPs on prescription.

Day Care

There are many different kinds of day care services organised locally either by social services or voluntary organisations. They can include luncheon clubs at day-centres, activities or trips out.

Home Helps and Home Care Assistants

Help in the home with household tasks and also with care needs. Precisely what tasks are undertaken varies locally.

Sitting Services and Respite Care

Both these types of services are designed to enable a carer to take a break, either by someone coming in to your home or giving the carer and the person cared for a break away from each other for a night, a day or longer.

Meals on Wheels

There are many different kinds of meals on wheels services, many run by voluntary organisations. Ask which days meals are delivered, whether they cater for special diets and charges and whether or not the meal is hot or frozen for reheating.

Laundry Services

Some special services departments run laundry services for people coping with incontinence or who cannot manage their laundry for other reasons.

Transport

Ambulances or care transport to day-care schemes, hospital appointments, luncheon clubs or outings.

Telephones, Communications and Alarms

These may be available from social services for telephone rental costs; special equipment may be available from British Telecom.

4 Who To Ask

There are lots of different people locally that may be a source of help, advice and assistance. Services may come from local voluntary organisations and a Citizen's Advice Bureau will be a good source of names and contact numbers. Alternatively the local Council for Voluntary Service or Community Health Council will have information about what is available locally. Some of the professionals you may need to get in touch with include social workers; district nurses; occupational therapists; physiotherapists; the community psychiatric nurse; your general practitioner.

Women's Royal Voluntary Service

omen's Royal Voluntary Service - or WRVS - has over 50 years' experience of providing care within the community. More than 150,000 members, including a growing number of men, give their time each year to help with family welfare, hospitals, food and emergency services. This means that WRVS is uniquely placed to meet the challenges and demands of an ever-changing society.

The nature of the work in which WRVS is involved means that training has an important role to play, so our volunteers have the opportunity to learn new skills, as well as making an important contribution to their local communites.

Emergency Services

isaster can strike at any time - a bomb explosion, train crash or flood. Wherever and whenever this happens, trained WRVS teams are called out to give help and comfort to victims. WRVS members are also on hand to provide support services for rescue workers.

Caring for Families

RVS has always been in the forefront of organising services and facilities which meet the real needs of the families. Today these include parent and toddler playgroups - a lifeline to young, isolated parents - toy libraries, family centres which provide much needed day care for young children and access centres for families going through the trauma of divorce. WRVS also works closely with offenders' families to help sustain family links during periods of separation.

Hospitals

RVS members are familiar figures in almost 900 hospitals throughout the country. They run shops for patients, staff and visitors, tea bars and ward trolleys, act as escorts, organise libraries, help

with flower arranging on wards and help with creches in ante-natal and other clinics.

Income-generating WRVS projects have an additional benefit as the profits are donated to the hospital to finance a wide variety of gifts such as medical equipment, refurbishment and amenities for patients and staff.

Organised Food Services

ome 70,000 volunteers are involved in delivering over 17 million meals a year through meals on wheels and luncheon clubs, ensuring housebound and elderly people can regularly enjoy hot, nourishing meals. WRVS offers either a complete cook and deliver service or delivery only.

WRVS pioneered the use of computers in organised food management and has developed a meals on wheels software package. This is used by several of the country's largest local authorities.

Changing to meet today's needs

ow, no less than in 1938 when WRVS was founded, a commitment to voluntary care in action remains at the heart of all our work. Like any large organisation, however, we recognise the importance of constant development so that we can continue with that commitment. Major changes in the way WRVS operates are now under way and these will provide a sure foundation for the future.

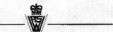

If you would like further information about WRVS or its caring services, please contact one of the offices listed overleaf, or check the local telephone directory for your nearest WRVS branch.

RESOURCE 1

*Greater London Council,
'Guidelines on Policy and
Practice Towards
Volunteers in Funded
Organisations', 1985*

The use of volunteers

1 The use of volunteers to provide a service is appropriate where:

a) It is important to consumers that the service-providers have a commitment to them which is not based on payment (for example, in some counselling services); or

b) The quality of the service depends on developing a personal relationship between consumers and service providers (for example, in befriending elderly people); or

c) It is important that consumers and service providers have shared similar experiences (for example, in mutual aid groups); and

d) Volunteers themselves benefit from their involvement (that is, in groups which have established good practice).

2 The use of volunteers is not appropriate where:

a) It is important that standards of services can be guaranteed (for example, in health care); or

b) It is important that levels of service can be guaranteed (for example, emergency services); or

c) They would substitute for statutory sector jobs which had been cut; or

d) They would threaten existing statutory sector jobs; or

e) They would threaten the terms and conditions of jobs in general.

3 Good practice

a) Organisations should extend equal opportunities practices to the recruitment of volunteers.

b) Volunteers should expect full reimbursement of out-of-pocket expenses. Procedures for claiming expenses should be accessible and easily understood.

c) Volunteers' involvement in decision-making should be as extensive as is possible.

d) Volunteers should be protected from marginalisation and should expect a varied and changing experience from their involvement, having regard to their abilities.

e) Volunteers should have equality of opportunity with paid staff for training, having regard to their separate roles within the organisations.

f) Volunteers should be insured in parity with paid employees.

g) Voluntary organisations have a responsibility to make volunteers aware of their rights within the organisation.

RESOURCE 9

*Carers National
Association,
'Carers Code'*

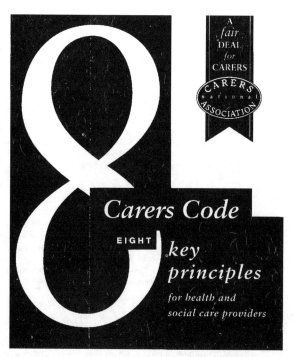

The Carers Code has been published by Carers National Association as part of their campaign, A Fair Deal for Carers.

A leaflet is available which explains the Fair Deal for Carers campaign and gives more information on Carers National Association. It is called 'Join the campaign for a Fair Deal for Carers'.

If you would like a copy of that leaflet, more information about the Code, or to share your ideas with us, please call 071-490 8818 or write to:

Carers National Association
20/25 Glasshouse Yard
London EC1A 4JS

Carers Code

EIGHT *key principles for health and social care providers*

We care because you do.

Carers Code

Eight key principles : a code of good practice for health and social care providers.

Most Community Care is provided by family, friends and relatives - the UK's seven million carers.

A great deal of progress has been made in recent years in recognising this contribution.

This Code sets out eight key principles which should be kept in mind when services for carers are being planned and delivered.

As well as the list of principles we give some examples of how they can be put into practice. We are sure many health and social care providers will be able to add examples from their own experience.

1 RECOGNITION

- of carers in their own right
- of their expertise and skill
- of their need for services

Turning the principle into practice:
- survey the numbers of carers in your area
- agree written policy statements eg definition of carer support services in Community Care plans
- use the media to reach out to 'hidden' carers
- be active in publicising services and support to carers

2 CHOICE

- about taking on the role of carer
- about whether to continue
- about how much and what care is provided

Turning the principle into practice:
Provide:
- honest information about what help is available
- counselling/advocacy services
- training for service providers
- good domiciliary care
- needs-led not service-driven care
- responsive and flexible services
- good alternatives to family care

3 EQUITY

Recognition of carers' individual needs, with regard to: • gender assumptions • cultural differences • age • sexual orientation • race • disability

Turning the principle into practice:

- equal opportunities training for staff
- services which don't discriminate
- information available in appropriate formats eg translated, jargon-free, in a variety of locations
- culturally sensitive services;
- monitor allocation and take up of services

4 CONSULTATION

- through representation
- through participation
- through acting on what you learn
- through developing the carers' voice

Turning the principle into practice:
- allocate staff time
- develop a variety of forms of consultation which is regularly reviewed
- invite carers onto committees
- provide funding for forums and relief care
- set up local carers projects
- give feedback, let people know

5 INFORMATION

- ensure all staff understand they have responsibility to signpost carers to appropriate information sources
- provide information before, during and after caring
- be open and honest

Turning the principle into practice:
- do outreach work, eg mobile buses
- use the media
- fund specific projects and workers
- provide multi-disciplinary training
- ensure regular information exchange between professionals
- set up help lines
- produce free directories and local information packs
- publicise your complaints procedure widely
- give clear information on charging policies

6 PROVISION OF PRACTICAL HELP

- assessment procedures which are speedy, well thought out and accessible
- develop specific **carer** focused services
- be flexible and provide services that carers want when they want them

Turning the principle into practice:
Provide:
- a separate assessment for carers
- weekend and evening sleep-in services
- services which allow carers to continue in paid employment
- family based respite
- transport
- more domestic help (eg cleaning, shopping)

7 MINIMISE THE COST OF CARING

- give information on benefits/help getting benefits
- agree policies which keep charges to a minimum

Turning the principle into practice:
- employ a carers' welfare rights worker
- provide benefits information in GPs' surgeries and hospitals
- agree charging policies which exclude disability benefits
- provide free temporary respite care
- assist carers to stay in paid employment

8 CO-ORDINATED SERVICES

- ensure service-providing agencies work together and communicate effectively
- ensure hospital discharge procedures involve carers at all stages
- involve voluntary and private sector agencies in planning and service development

Turning the principle into practice:
- provide multi-disciplinary assessments
- ensure agreement from patients and carers about hospital discharge procedures
- review how discharge procedures are working
- appoint a 'named person' to co-ordinate care package
- ensure primary health care teams understand local assessment procedure and refer appropriately
- set up regular inter-agency meetings and shared training

RESOURCE 10

Mary Ryan,
The Guardian,
20 July, 1988

A last civil rights battle

Rachel Hurst, chair of Greenwich Association of Disabled People, calls it 'the last civil rights movement'. Over the past decade, the anger, energy and momentum of the disability movement has brought a proliferation of associations set up and controlled by disabled people.

Mainstream charities and agencies, say these groups, have failed to devolve power sufficiently to disabled people or to involve them in designing the services they will eventually use. Out of this has arisen a dichotomy between organisations of – controlled by – disabled people, and organisations for them, which generally have the able-bodied acting on their behalf.

At national level, the 'ofs' affiliate with the British Council of Organisations of Disabled People (BCODP) and the 'fors' with the Royal Association for Disability and Rehabilitation (RADAR). Internationally, BCODP is affiliated to Disabled Peoples' International (DPI), the association of organisations controlled by disabled people, and RADAR to Rehabilitation International, which has been notorious for its reluctance to transfer control.

Bert Massie, RADAR's assistant director of disablement services, argues that there is a lot more cross-fertilisation between 'fors' and 'ofs' than the disabled allow. While crediting BCODP with raising issues of disabled people's empowerment, he suggests that institutions like the Spastics Society and Royal National Institute for the Blind are working towards the same goals, and have many disabled people at senior level.

Yet financial disparities cause some bitterness. Although BCODP represents 43 organisations of disabled people throughout the country, and though its membership of DPI is recognised by the United Nations as their national representative voice, it receives only £10,000 annually in government funding. RADAR gets around £250,000.

Richard Wood, who chairs BCODP, says, 'The British Government has not afforded BCODP the same status as RADAR – an unrepresentative body – even though the Government is a signatory to UN Resolution 37/152, which says member nations should increase assistance to organisations of disabled people and help them to organise and co-ordinate the representation of their interests and concerns.'

The chief theoretical arm of the disability movement is the Union of Physically Impaired Against Segregation (UPIAS), formed in 1974. Vic Finkelstein, a founder member who currently runs an Open University course on The Handicapped Person In The Community, traces the origins of disability to society rather than perceiving it as merely an individual problem needing individual solutions.

Buildings, technical aids and transport are all geared to the needs of able-bodied people; so 'disability' is imposed by the way society is organised and additional to physical impairment rather than inherent in it. With well chosen technical aids, care attendance support, appropriate housing, transport and workplaces, 'disability' can be markedly diminished. This model of disability as a form of social oppression is now widely accepted.

Aspirations towards 'normality' are rejected for implying that it is the disabled person who has to change, not society. 'I'm proud of being a disabled person', says Rachel Hurst. 'I don't want to be cured. Cured of what? I feel comfortable with what I am, even though I feel angry when I can't do in life what I would like to do because of social attitudes and barriers.'

Finkelstein points to occupational therapy as one area where token moves have been made towards working more in partnership with disabled people, but feels this is too little, too late.

'The contradictions are sharpening up. Disabled people want less and less people doing things for them and, as the Centres for Integrated Living are being set up, they're appreciating that they can do even that kind of job better. There really is a revolution going on. Most professionals don't understand it. They have no information about this movement because it is outside their professional experience.'

There are now five Centres for Independent Living (CILS) in Britain, with a further two being developed. Like the American CILs, which provided much of the initial inspiration, they are local, non-residential centres which offer support and services under the direct control of disabled people.

The Derbyshire Coalition of Disabled People took its first steps towards setting up a CIL in 1981 and with over 30 employees it is now the largest in the country. Seven areas were outlined as crucial to disabled people's empowerment and integration: information, counselling, suitably designed housing, appropriate technical aids, personal assistance, transport and access. The CIL offers practical assistance and advice in all seven.

While the American model emphasised the need for disabled people themselves to provide services, the Derbyshire Coalition felt that local needs would be better served by involving able-bodied workers as well. To reflect the different emphasis, the Derbyshire CIL is known as a Centre for Integrated Living.

'We could see that the idea of a Centre for Independent Living would be very attractive to a Thatcherite government', says Ken Davis, former chair of the Coalition, 'and there was no wish to lend ourselves as a convenient vehicle for the dismantling of the welfare state. The coalition's basic view was that any civilised social response to the needs of physically impaired people should be collectively underwritten.

'But at the same time we wanted to get rid of that form of welfarism based on the perception of people as passive recipients. That had to be challenged'.

The Derbyshire CIL works with, and is financed by, statutory bodies, and acts as 'a persuasive voice' in local authority decisions. The political pressure work has been kept separate from service provision, with the coalition doing the first and the CIL the second.

The principles underpinning the much smaller Greenwich CIL are very similar. Transport and access were identified as particularly important if disabled people were to get together to fight for their rights.

'We can't effect change until we become part of the political arena', says Rachel Hurst, 'and we can't become part of the political arena until we have access to social structures at all levels, until we can get out of our homes, and out of the institutions in which we've been incarcerated. Greenwich still has many hundreds, maybe thousands, of disabled people who still can't move around their own homes, use their own toilets, use their own bedrooms and even get in and out of their own houses. We've still got a long way to go.'

There are CILs in Derbyshire, Greenwich, Hampshire, Southampton and Nottingham, with others being developed in Strathclyde and Milton Keynes.

REFERENCES

ABBOTT, P. and WALLACE, C. (1990) 'Women's work' in *An Introduction to Sociology: Feminist perspectives*, Routledge.

ABRAMS, P. (1977) 'Community care: some research problems and priorities', *Policy and Politics*, 6 (2): 125–151.

ACKERS, H. L. (1985) *The Provision of Day-Centres for Elderly Members of Ethnic Minorities*, Greater London Council.

ACKERS, H. L. (1986) *Evaluation of the Trefgarne Initiative: Report to Social Services Committee*, Avon County Council.

ACKERS, H. L. *et al.* (1989) *Unmet Needs and the Disabled Person's Act*, Report to West Devon Social Services Committee, July.

ANDREWS, K. (1984) 'Private rest homes in the care of the elderly', *British Medical Journal*, 288: 1518–1520.

ANDREWS, K. and JACOBS, J. (1990) *Punishing the Poor: Poverty under Thatcher*, Macmillan.

AUDIT COMMISSION (1986) *Making a Reality of Community Care*, HMSO.

BAYLEY, R. (1993) 'House that tax built', *The Guardian*, October 15: 21.

BBC (1991) *Getting the Social and Health Care You Need. Take Care: You and Yours Factsheet*, BBC.

BECKER, S. *et al.* (1993) *Who Cares in Nottinghamshire?*, Department of Social Sciences, Loughborough University.

BECKER, S. (1995) 'Poverty and social welfare' in Caterrall, P. (ed.) (1995) *Contemporary Britain: An annual review 1995*, Institute of Contemporary British History.

BLACK REPORT (1980): *see* Department of Health & Social Security (1980).

BRENTON, M. (1985) *The Voluntary Sector in British Social Services*, Longman.

BRINDLE, D. (1993a) 'North–South health divide "widening"', *The Guardian*, November 15: 4.

BRINDLE, D. (1993b) 'Funding famine strands users of wheelchairs', *The Guardian*, 11 October: 5.

BRINDLE, D. (1994a) 'Firms cut cash gifts to charity', *The Guardian*, 23 May: 2.

BRINDLE, D. (1994b) 'Friends in need', *The Guardian, Society*, 26 January: 15.

BRINDLE, D. (1994c) 'Rich cup or poison chalice?', *The Guardian, Society*, 18 May: 12–13.

BRITISH HEART FOUNDATION (1994) *Coronary Heart Disease Statistics. 1993 Edition*, British Heart Foundation/Coronary Prevention Group Statistics Database.

BRITISH MEDICAL JOURNAL (1986) 'Lies, damned lies and suppressed statistics', Editorial, *British Medical Journal*, 293: 349–350.

BROWN, M. (1990) *Introduction to Social Administration in Britain* (7th edn), Hutchinson University Library Press.

BULMER, M. *et al.* (1989) 'The goals of social policy: Part IV' in *Social Policy and the Community*, Unwin Hyman.

CARERS NATIONAL ASSOCIATION (1993) *Young Carers*, CNA.

CARERS NATIONAL ASSOCIATION (1994a) *Facts About Carers*, 23 (IS), CNA.

CARERS NATIONAL ASSOCIATION (1994b) *Carers Code: Eight key principles for health and social care providers*, CNA.

CENTRAL STATISTICAL OFFICE (1993a) *Social Trends 23*, HMSO.

CENTRAL STATISTICAL OFFICE (1993b) *Regional Trends 28*, HMSO.

CENTRAL STATISTICAL OFFICE (1994a) *Social Trends 24*, HMSO.

CENTRAL STATISTICAL OFFICE (1994b) *Family Spending: A report on the 1993 Family Expenditure Survey,* HMSO.

CENTRAL STATISTICAL OFFICE (1994c) *Annual Abstract of Statistics 1993, No. 129*, HMSO.

COMMISSION FOR RACIAL EQUALITY (1994) *Race Relations Code of Practice for Maternity Services,* CRE.

CONSERVATIVE PARTY (1992) *The Best Future for Britain: The Conservative manifesto 1992*, Conservative Central Office.

DALLEY, G. (1988) *Ideologies of Caring,* Macmillan.

DAVIS, A. (1993) 'Community care' in Spurgeon, P. (ed.) (1993) *The New Face of the NHS*, Longman.

DEPARTMENT OF THE ENVIRONMENT (1993) *English House Condition Survey 1991*, HMSO.

DEPARTMENT OF HEALTH & SOCIAL SECURITY (1976) *Sharing Resources for Health in England: Report of the Resource Allocation Working Party*, HMSO.

DEPARTMENT OF HEALTH & SOCIAL SECURITY (1980) *Inequalities in Health: Report of a Research Working Group* [Chairman: Sir Douglas Black], DHSS.

DEPARTMENT OF HEALTH & SOCIAL SECURITY (1983) *NHS Management Inquiry* [Chairman: Mr (later Sir) Roy Griffiths], DA (83) 38, DHSS.

DEPARTMENT OF HEALTH (1989a) *Working for Patients*, HMSO.

DEPARTMENT OF HEALTH (1989b) *Caring for People: Community care in the next decade and beyond*, Cmnd. 849, HMSO.

DEPARTMENT OF HEALTH (1991a) *The Patient's Charter: Raising the standard*, HMSO.

DEPARTMENT OF HEALTH (1991b) *The Health of the Nation: A consultative document for health in England*, Cmnd. 1523, HMSO.

DEPARTMENT OF HEALTH (1992) *The Health of the Nation: A strategy for health in England*, Cmnd. 1986, HMSO.

DEPARTMENT OF HEALTH SOCIAL SERVICES INSPECTORATE (1991) *Purchase of Service: Practice guidance and practice material for social services departments and other agencies*, HMSO.

DINGWALL, R. (1979) 'Inequality and the National Health Service', in Atkinson, P., Dingwall, R. and Murcott, A. (1979) *Prospects for the National Health*, Croom Helm.

DONNISON, D. (1994) 'Riches to die for', *The Guardian, Society*, 27 July: 12–13.

DOWLING, S. (1983) *Health for a Change: The provision of preventive health care in pregnancy and early childhood*, Child Poverty Action Group/National Extension College.

EATON, L. (1993) 'Open to abuse', *Nursing Times*, 89 (44): 16.

ELLIOTT, L. and KELLY, R. (1994) 'Tories' £125-a-month boost for the rich', *The Guardian*, 9 February: 7.

EQUAL OPPORTUNITIES COMMISSION (1982) *Who Cares for the Carers? Opportunities for those caring for the elderly and handicapped*, EOC.

EQUAL OPPORTUNITIES COMMISSION (1984) *Carers and Services: A comparison of men and women caring for dependent elderly people*, EOC.

FINCH, J. and GROVES, D. (eds) (1983) *A Labour of Love: Women, work and caring*, Routledge & Kegan Paul.

FINKELSTEIN, V. (1980) *Attitudes and Disabled People: Issues for discussion*, World Rehabilitation Fund.

FITZPATRICK, B. and TAYLOR, R. (1994a) 'A comparative study of quality criteria', *Nursing Standard*, 8 (37): 25–29.

FITZPATRICK, B. and TAYLOR, R. (1994b) 'Patients' criteria in assessing quality', *Nursing Standard*, 8 (38): 34–39.

FOX, A. J. and LEON, D. A. (1985) *Mortality and Deprivation: Evidence from the OPCS Longitudinal Study*, Working Paper 33, Social Statistics Research Unit, The City University.

FRIES, R. (1994) 'But is it in the public interest?', *The Guardian, Society*, 22 June: 10–11.

GARRETT, G. (1990) *Older People: Their support and care*, Macmillan.

GENERAL SYNOD OF THE CHURCH OF ENGLAND (1985) *Faith in the City*, Church House Publishing.

GINSBURG, N. (1993) *Divisions of Welfare*, Sage.

GOFFMAN, E. (1968) *Asylums*, Doubleday and Co., New York.

GRAHAM, H. (1984) *Health and Welfare*, Macmillan.

GREAT BRITAIN: Inter-departmental Committee on Social Insurance and Allied Services (1942) *Social Insurance and Allied Services: Report* [Chairman: W. K. Beveridge], Cmnd. 6404, HMSO.

GREAT BRITAIN: Social Services Committee (1980) *Perinatal and Neonatal Mortality: Second Report, 1979–1980* [Chair: Mrs Renee Short], HMSO.

GREAT BRITAIN: Standing Maternity and Midwifery Advisory Committee (1970) *Domiciliary Midwifery and Maternity Bed Needs* [Chairman: J. Peel], HMSO.

GREATER LONDON COUNCIL (1985) *Guidelines on Policy and Practice Towards Volunteers in Funded Organisations*, GLC.

GREEN, H. (1990) *Informal Carers* (General Household Survey 1985, GHS 15, Supplement A), Office of Population Censuses and Surveys.

GRIFFITHS, Sir R. (1988) *Community Care: An agenda for action. A report to the Secretary of State for Social Services*, HMSO.

HARMAN, H. (1993) 'Portillo's poor pillars of principle', *The Guardian*, 27 October: 24.

HEALY, P. (1993) 'Arrangements for care', *Nursing Times*, 89 (3): 26–29.

HILL, M. (1990) *Social Security Policy in Britain*, Edward Elgar, Aldershot.

HUNT, S. *et al.* (1986) 'Housing and health in a deprived area of Edinburgh', paper presented to the Institute of Environmental Health Officers/Legal Research Institute conference on 'Unhealthy housing: a diagnosis' at Warwick University, 14–16 December 1986.

ILLSLEY, R. (1986) 'Occupational class, selection and the production of inequalities in health', *Quarterly Journal of Social Affairs*, 2 (2): 151–165.

INSTITUTE FOR PUBLIC POLICY RESEARCH (1994) *Social Justice: Strategies for national renewal*, IPPR.

JAMIESON, A. (1991) 'Community care for older people: policies in Britain, West Germany and Denmark' in Room, G. (ed.) (1991) *Towards a European Welfare State*, SAUS.

JOHNSON, N. (1990) 'Problems for the mixed economy of welfare' in Ware, A. and Goodin, E. (eds) (1990) *Needs and Welfare*, Sage Publications.

JOHNSON, P. (1989) 'Old age creeps up', *Marxism Today*, January: 34–39.

JONES, K. and FOWLES, A. (1983) 'People in institutions: rhetoric and reality' in Jones, C. and Stevenson, J. (1983) *Yearbook of Social Policy in Britain*, Routledge.

JOSEPH ROWNTREE FOUNDATION (1995) *Inquiry into Income and Wealth*, Vols. I and II, Joseph Rowntree Foundation.

JOSEPH ROWNTREE MEMORIAL TRUST (1992) 'Household budgets and living standards', *Social Policy Research Findings*, 31, November, Joseph Rowntree Memorial Trust.

KEMPSON, E., BRYSON, A. and ROWLINGSON, K. (1994) *Hard Times? How poor families make ends meet*, Policy Studies Institute.

KENDALL, S. and McANULTY, L. (1990) *Inequalities in Health and the Provision of Care*, Distance Learning Centre, South Bank University.

KINGMAN, S. (1994) 'Community care: the first year. Newcastle: making strides', *British Medical Journal* (308): 966–969.

KNIGHT, B. (1993) *Voluntary Action*, Home Office on behalf of Centris.

LABOUR PARTY (1992) *Better Community Care: Labour's policies for improving care in the community*, The Labour Party.

LABOUR PARTY (1994) *Health 2000: The health and wealth of the nation*, The Labour Party.

LAING & BUISSON (1993) *Laing's Review of Private Healthcare 1993*, Laing & Buisson.

LEAT, D. (1987) *Voluntary Organisations and Accountability: Theory and practice*, University of Warwick.

LE GRAND, J. (1982) *The Strategy of Equality*, Allen & Unwin.

LONSDALE, S. (1990) *Women and Disability*, Macmillan Education.

LYNCH, P. and OELMAN, B. J. (1981) 'Mortality from coronary heart disease in the British Army compared with the civil population', *British Medical Journal*, 283: 405–407.

McKEOWN, T. (1976) *The Modern Rise of Population and the Role of Medicine: Dream, mirage or nemesis?*, Rock Karling Monograph, Nuffield Provincial Hospitals Trust.

MACK, J. and LANSLEY, S. (1985) *Poor Britain*, Allen & Unwin.

MARMOT, M. G., SHIPLEY, M. J. and ROSE, G. (1984) 'Inequalities in death: specific explanations of a general pattern', *The Lancet*, 2 (8384): 1003–1006.

MARMOT, M. G. and McDOWALL, M. E. (1986) 'Mortality decline and widening social inequalities', *The Lancet*, 2 (8501): 274–276.

MARR, J. and KHADIM, N. (1994) 'Meeting the needs of ethnic patients', *Nursing Standard*, 8 (3): 31–33.

MARSH, A. and McKAY, S. (1994) *Poor Smokers*, Policy Studies Institute.

MARSH, G. N. and CHANNING, D. M. (1986) 'Deprivation and health in one general practice', *British Medical Journal*, 292: 1173–1176.

MEREDITH, B. (1993) *The Community Care Handbook: The new system explained*, Age Concern.

MERRETT, S. (1979) *State Housing in Britain*, Routledge & Kegan Paul.

MINISTRY OF HEALTH (1944) *White Paper on a National Health Service*, HMSO.

MOHAN, J. (1991) 'Privatisation in the British health sector: a challenge to the NHS?', in Gabe, J., Calnan, M. and Bury, M. (eds) (1991) *The Sociology of the Health Service*, Routledge.

MORRIS, J. K., COOK, D. G. and SHAPER, A. G. (1994) 'Loss of employment and mortality', *British Medical Journal*, 308: 1135–1139.

MURRAY, C. (ed.) (1990) *The Emerging British Underclass*, Institute for Economic Affairs.

MURRAY, C. (1994) 'The underclass deepens', *The Sunday Times*, 22 May.

MUSCULAR DYSTROPHY GROUP (1993) *Batteries Not Included*, MDG.

NISSELL, M. and BONNERJEA, L. (1982) *Family Care of the Handicapped Elderly: Who pays?*, Policy Studies Institute.

NOLAN, M. and GRANT, G. (1989) 'Addressing the needs of informal carers: a neglected area of practice, *Journal of Advanced Nursing*, 14: 950–961.

NURSING TIMES (1993) 'Carers want better respite services', *Nursing Times*, 89 (50): 9.

OLIVER, M. (1983) *Social Work with Disabled People*, Macmillan.

OLIVER, M. (1990) *The Politics of Disablement*, Macmillan Education.

OORSCHOT, W. V. (1991) 'Non-take-up of social security benefits in Europe', *Journal of European Social Policy*, 1 (1):15–30.

OFFICE OF POPULATION CENSUSES AND SURVEYS (1986) *Registrar General's Decennial Supplement on Occupational Mortality 1979–83*, HMSO.

OFFICE OF POPULATION CENSUSES AND SURVEYS (1992) *General Household Survey 1990*, GHS 22, HMSO.

OFFICE OF POPULATION CENSUSES AND SURVEYS (1993a) *General Household Survey 1991*, GHS 23, HMSO.

OFFICE OF POPULATION CENSUSES AND SURVEYS (1993b) *Health Survey for England 1991*, HMSO.

PARKER, G. (1985) *With Due Care and Attention. A review of research on informal care*, Family Policy Studies Centre.

PENDLETON, D. A. and BOCHNER, S. (1980) 'The communication of medical information in general practice consultations as a function of patients' social class', *Social Science and Medicine*, 14: 669–673.

PHILLIMORE, P., BEATTIE, A. and TOWNSEND, P. (1994) 'Widening inequality of health in northern England, 1981–91', *British Medical Journal*, 308: 1125–1128.

PHOENIX, A. (1990) 'Black women and the maternity services' in Garcia, J., Kilpatrick, R. and Richards, M. (eds) (1990) *The Politics of Maternity Care*, Clarendon Press.

PITKEATHLEY, J. (1991) 'Caring concerns', *Nursing Times*, 87 (34): 24.

PITKEATHLEY, J. (1992) 'A voice for an unsung army', *Care of the Elderly*, 4 (10): 444–445.

POLICY STUDIES INSTITUTE (1993) *Families, Work and Benefits*, Policy Studies Institute.

POLLOCK, A. (1994) 'Carers' literature review', *Nursing Times*, 90 (25): 31–33.

RANADE, W. (1994) *A Future for the NHS? Health care in the 1990s*. Longman.

READING, R., COLVER, A., OPENSHAW, S. and JARVIS, S. (1994) 'Do interventions that improve immunisation uptake also reduce social inequalities in uptake?', *British Medical Journal*, 308: 1142–1144.

RYAN, M. (1988) 'A last civil rights battle', *The Guardian*, 20 July.

SMITH, S. (1993) 'All change', *Nursing Times*, 89 (3): 24–26.

SOCIAL SERVICES COMMITTEE (1980): see Great Britain.

STEVENS, A. (1991) *Disability Issues: Developing anti-discriminatory practice*, CCETSW.

TAWNEY, R. H. (1981) *Equality*, Allen & Unwin.

TAYLOR-GOOBY, P. (1989) 'Disquiet and welfare: clinging to Nanny', *International Journal of Urban and Regional Research*, 13: 201–216.

TITMUSS, R. M. (1955) 'The social division of welfare' in *Essays on the Welfare State*, Allen & Unwin.

TITMUSS, R. M. (1968) *Commitment to Welfare*, Allen & Unwin.

TITMUSS, R. M. (1973) *The Gift Relationship*, Penguin.

TIZARD, J. (ed.) (1975) *Varieties of Residential Experience*, Routledge & Kegan Paul.

TOWNSEND, P. (1962) *The Last Refuge*, Routledge & Kegan Paul.

TOWNSEND, P. (1979) *Poverty in the UK*, Penguin.

TOWNSEND, P. and DAVIDSON, N. (eds) (1988) 'The Black Report' in Townsend, P., Davidson, N. and Whitehead, M. (1992) *Inequalities in Health: The Black Report* and *The Health Divide* (rev. edn), Penguin.

TOWNSEND, P., PHILLIMORE, P. and BEATTIE, A. (1988) *Health and Deprivation: Inequality in the North*, Croom Helm.

TUDOR HART, J. (1971) 'The inverse care law', *The Lancet*, 1.

UNIVERSITY OF PLYMOUTH (1993) *Equal Opportunities Policy*, University of Plymouth.

WAINE, B. (1992) 'The voluntary sector: the Thatcher years' in Manning, N. and Page, R. (eds), *Social Policy Review 4*, Social Policy Association.

WARE, A. (1991) 'Meeting needs through voluntary action: does market society corrode altruism?' in Ware, A. and Goodin, R. E. (1991) *Needs and Welfare*, Sage Publications.

WARE, A. and GOODIN, R. E. (1991) *Needs and Welfare*, Sage Publications.

WARNER, N. (1994) *Community Care: Just a fairy tale?*, Carers National Association.

WEST, P. (1984) 'The family, the welfare state and community care: political rhetoric and public attitudes', *Journal of Social Policy*, 13 (4): 417–446.

WHITE, M. (1993) 'English NHS managers up 262pc', *The Guardian*, 18 November: 3.

WHITEHEAD, M. (1988) 'The health divide' in Townsend, P., Davidson, N. and Whitehead, M. (1992) *Inequalities in Health: The Black Report* and *The Health Divide* (rev. edn), Penguin.

WHITEHEAD, M. (1994) 'Who cares about equity in the NHS?', *British Medical Journal*, 308: 1284–1287.

WILKINSON, R. (1994) *Unfair Shares: The effects of widening income differences on the welfare of the young*, Barnardo's.

WILLMOTT, P. (1986) *Social Networks, Informal Care and Public Policy*, Policy Studies Institute.

WILLMOTT, P. and THOMAS, D. (1984) *Community in Social Policy*, Policy Studies Institute.

WINTOUR, P. (1993) 'Portillo conjures up Christian lessons for welfare cutback', *The Guardian*, 16 September: 24.

WOMEN'S ROYAL VOLUNTARY SERVICE (1992) *Caring for Thousands*, WRVS.

WOOD, P. (1981) *International Classification of Impairments, Disabilities and Handicaps*, World Health Organization: Geneva.

WOOLLEY, F. and LE GRAND, J. (1990) 'The Ackroyds, the Osbornes and the Welfare State: The impact of the welfare state on two hypothetical families over their life-times', *Policy and Politics*, 18 (1): 17–30.

WORLD HEALTH ORGANIZATION (1985) *Targets for Health for All: The health policy for Europe*, WHO Regional Office for Europe, Copenhagen.

YOUNG, B. (1980) 'Health and housing: infestation', *Roof*, July–August 1980: 111–112.

YOUNG, P. (1989) *Mastering Social Welfare*, Macmillan.